what works for bipolar kids

what works for bipolar kids

HELP AND HOPE FOR PARENTS

Mani Pavuluri, MD, PhD

Foreword by Susan Resko, MM

THE GUILFORD PRESS
New York   London

Library of Congress Cataloging-in-Publication Data

Pavuluri, Mani N.
    What works for bipolar kids : help and hope for parents / by Mani Pavuluri.
          p.   cm.
    Includes bibliographical references and index.
    ISBN: 978-1-59385-407-2 (pbk. : alk. paper)
    ISBN: 978-1-59385-706-6 (hardcover : alk. paper)
    1. Manic–depressive illness in children—Popular works.
I. Title.
    RJ506.D4P38 2008
    618.92'895—dc22

                                                    2008002168

Contents

PART III
Pulling It All Together into Strategies for Specific Situations: Wisdom That Gets You Centered

APPENDICES

Foreword

When I was asked to write the foreword for *What Works for Bipolar Kids*, I was thrilled. I've known Mani Pavuluri for several years through her participation on the Child and Adolescent Bipolar Foundation (CABF) Professional Advisory Council and more recently as my son's child psychiatrist. Dr. Pavuluri's warmth and optimism, combined with her stature as one of the world's leading pediatric bipolar disorder researchers, make her an ideal expert to provide parents with information, support, and hope.

Raising a child with bipolar disorder is one of the most difficult challenges a parent can experience. Like juvenile diabetes, bipolar disorder is more severe when it first occurs in childhood. The disorder ravages children's growing brains as they struggle to make sense of their world while being pummeled by rapidly whipsawing emotions, thoughts, and energy levels. Parents not only must mourn the loss of an idyllic childhood, but also may experience physical and verbal abuse from their child, reprimands from friends and family who think the child just needs more love or discipline or routine or (you fill in the blank), doubts from clinicians who don't *believe in* child-onset bipolar disorder (as if it were a religion), judgmental comments from strangers in the grocery store, and questions from school personnel inquiring, "What is happening at home?" When a child suffers from cancer, friends and family circle the wagons with love and support, but when a child has bipolar disorder, parents are lost and alone on the wild frontier.

As a parent of a child with bipolar disorder, you never know what kind of person will greet you in the morning: one with unbounded energy and excitement or an anguished and intensely miserable child. And that's just the beginning of the day! That person who woke up in the morning may change several times throughout the day, and you must help navigate your child's rollercoaster emotions while trying to maintain stability and balance for the rest of your household.

It is for these reasons, and many more, that Dr. Pavuluri's book is a lifeline for parents raising children with bipolar disorder. Her genuine affection for children, combined with her superior knowledge and her glass-is-half-full outlook, provides parents with the right tools to help their children attain the highest level of wellness. Dr. Pavuluri's warm and enthusiastic personality comes alive in the book and offers encouragement for parents. Even though the treatment course is complicated for this serious illness, children with bipolar disorder can get better. Dr. Pavuluri charts a roadmap to success, or, as she would say, a rainbow of hope.

During my 6 years at CABF, I have heard heartbreaking and painful stories from parents who have all but lost hope; tales of untreated children and teens so intensely unstable, irritable, and tormented that they are ravaging their homes and destroying their family life. When a child is newly diagnosed with bipolar disorder, parents are faced with an overwhelming number of challenges. Chief among these is the need for a knowledgeable treatment team, education, resources, and support. Dr. Pavuluri teaches parents how to meet and even defeat these challenges.

As a parent of a child with bipolar disorder, the heart-wrenching stories I hear at CABF echo my own personal experience. My son suffered for years until we were able to find a treatment team that was knowledgeable and experienced enough to truly help him. My son has been so very fortunate to be under the care of Dr. Pavuluri; she has provided him with a higher level of wellness for which I barely dared to hope and dream.

I have always striven to help my son attain the next level of wellness, to take another step toward attaining a fulfilling and happy life. Many brilliant philosophers, artists, and political leaders lived with bipolar disorder. For the past decade, I relentlessly endeavored to help my son control the horrible illness symptoms so that his talents and gifts could shine. I was constantly seeking ways to minimize his symptoms so that his skills could be revealed, instead of appreciating the boy I was living with each day. Like many other parents of severely ill children, the role of case manager was threatening to consume me and my relationship with my son.

What I find most wonderful about Dr. Pavuluri is her ability to help me set *realistic* expectations for my son and to help our family look on the bright side of life, despite the severe illness that is always lurking in the shadows and periodically rears its ugly head. Under her care, we are learning to find acceptance for this devastating illness. She helps parents of children with bipolar disorder find the joy in parenting again, the joy that has been lost to so many. Dr. Pavuluri helps parents do all that her research and proven methods have revealed, but then sit back and find grace and happiness again, even in the face of the ever-approaching storm.

I hope you will enjoy this book as much as I did, not just for the critical information Dr. Pavuluri's expertise provides, but also for the optimism and hope she conveys—hope for a brighter future, but at the same time hope that you will find happiness today even in the face of a horrible illness.

SUSAN RESKO, MM
Executive Director
Child and Adolescent Bipolar Foundation

Acknowledgments

I wrote this book for parents and caregivers of bipolar children and also for youth who suffer from mood swings that look almost like bipolar disorder. These children are suffering silently on the inside, unable to find the words to articulate their emotional pain and searing distress, unable to manage relationships or be insightful while manic. Parents, as much as they understand their kids and love them desperately, are frequently miserable. I am bombarded with e-mails, phone calls, and letters with cries for help, some from places so far away—so many that I cannot answer them all in person. I know there are many good books out there, but I wanted to write about these kids my way, to talk directly to parents the way I do in my clinic. The compassion I felt for these children with bipolar disorder and related mood disorders and their parents and clinicians is what urged me to write this book. They taught me what bipolar disorder feels like. When I was lucky enough to have the chance to treat them, I got to see how it felt to have overcome this illness. They taught me that there is a bright light at the end of the tunnel. I want everyone to see that bright light. So, thank you to all the children, parents, and clinicians— you're the magnificent force behind this book.

I would like to thank Dr. Patrick Tolan, director of our Institute for Juvenile Research, who gave me the full freedom to design and develop my clinical and research programs to serve children with mood disorders, without which I would not have realized my dreams of helping these children. Dr. John Sweeney, my beloved mentor and friend, gave me the energy and resilience to tackle the most critical problems in researching these special children—he is a giant source of strength each day. Dean

Joseph Flaherty at the University of Illinois at Chicago College of Medicine is my cheerleader every step of the way—I feel so fortunate to have such great leadership behind me.

Then I have my team of gold that taught me the qualities that are essential to treat these children: persistence, patience, and endurance. I have to single out Dr. Julie Carbray, whom I call my soul sister. She serves as administrative director for the clinic and shares the craft of treating these children with me. She helped me write about health insurance coverage in this book. Drs. Amy West, Tahseen Mohammed, and David Henry and Mrs. Jodi Heidenreich are all amazing people who gave me ideas and showed me what first-class therapy looks like! This book took shape from the magic of our team. My program coordinator-cum-assistant, Anne Palmer, tirelessly typed my dictations for this book at lightning speed.

I feel the deepest gratitude for the extraordinary commitment of Doug and Margey Colbeth for sharing their strife and for their philanthropy in supporting our programs and deepening my commitment to delivering nothing but the very best to families. They are my guideposts. This book is in part an effort to pay tribute to them by striving for my goals.

How could I have ever finished the book without the help of Deborah Popely, with her extraordinary talent for changing my Indian English to proper English and stringing my dictations into this current shape? It would have been impossible to write this book without her utter dedication to the details as she developed a deep relationship with the topic. The heart and soul of this book is my editor, Chris Benton, who carefully crafted the chapters and has drawn out the boxes of tips to offer the gist of the ideas at their best to readers. I really felt that it was just like listening to a beautiful piece of music when I looked at her tracked corrections or comments. Her highly insightful and gorgeous e-mails gave me the momentum I needed to finish the book that competed with many grant- and paper-writing projects over 2 years. Without her, there would be no book. Chris, you are my ultimate star. Kitty Moore, Executive Editor at The Guilford Press, needless to say, is the overarching force and guide behind the team that had the vision for us to do this book. Thanks also to Dr. Peter Jensen, who recruited me to write the book for Guilford, and Dr. Gaye Carlson, who believed that I could. I am indebted to Anna Brackett for the immaculate effort required to bring the manuscript into its final form.

Susan Resko, the Executive Director of the Child and Adolescent Bipolar Foundation (CABF), is a dear friend and the engine behind the enrichment of this book with the voices of parents. Thanks also to Nanci Schiman, who runs CABF's parent-to-parent support program and gathered and organized the touching quotes from CABF members. Thanks to all those parents who breathed life into the narration. Susan's meticulous suggestions were priceless. CABF's efforts were supported by a grant for this book from the van Ameringen Foundation, for which I am very grateful. Susan Berger with the Blue Harbor Foundation has also inspired me with a parent's voice that was precious.

I am thankful for the unconditional love and affection that my parents gave me that stands as a well-founded model for my thoughts. I consider myself incredibly lucky that my mom gave me an appreciation for the polarity of deep emotions through bedtime stories such as *Hamlet* and *The Comedy of Errors* at a very early age. My darling husband, Naren, never ever complains about my spending hours and hours on my laptop, as while working on this book. I admire him each time he says, "Do what is important and makes a difference." We have two absolutely delightful and spunky boys, Rohan and Chetan, who crack me up with laughter and completely bring me down to earth with the humility of parenthood. They keep me grounded and teach me lessons in how to be a good mom. I will never forget the moment when they ran to get me something to eat at 1:00 A.M. in the New Delhi Airport while I was typing away on this book, and tried to catch my attention by turning my face to them, holding my cheeks with their little hands. Thank you, big guys!

Helping Your Bipolar Child

A FRESH OUTLOOK

If you have a child with bipolar disorder, every day may feel a little like riding a wild horse. You don't know where the day will take you or how you and your child will emerge from the experience. And just when you think you've gotten the situation in hand, it kicks up its heels and blindsides you. You may not know what else you can do to control the mood swings, and you worry about the future of your bipolar child and your family.

This book is about taming bipolar disorder so that your child and your family can lead the lives you were meant to have. It's about learning a new set of principles and adopting a toolbox full of strategies that will give you a fresh approach to getting through the day when you feel like the only thing you can expect is the unexpected. It's about helping your child *and* your family (and, yes, even yourself). Most of all it's about hope, and knowing, as one mother put it so eloquently, that "staying hopeful is all about remembering that your child is really that sweet innocent blessing of a being that you would give your very life for."

I have been working with children who have bipolar disorder and their families for more than 20 years, and, naturally, one of the very first questions parents ask me is "Will my child ever get better?" Invariably, my answer is "There is an excellent chance, but we need to work toward it." Whether you're in the midst of exploring the possibility that your child has bipolar disorder, just received a diagnosis, or are already coping with the diagnosis on a daily basis, a positive, happy, and successful future for your child may seem like a lot to hope for. But my experience has shown that it's possible when you have the right tools.

The purpose of this book is to offer you those tools. I have assembled this tool kit from my years of work with bipolar children at our Pediatric Mood Disorders Program at the University of Illinois at Chicago. There, my colleagues and I explore brain function in children and teens with mood disorders in our neuroscience research laboratory, study treatments that help regulate moods in our treatment development lab, and serve families in a multidisciplinary clinic. Through this combination of treating children, working with their families, and conducting research, we learn more every day about the best possible ways to help children who have bipolar disorder. We've made encouraging strides: 68% of the children and adolescents were stabilized over 18 months following the medication approach we've developed. And, with the help of a very specific type of psychotherapy, we've seen these improvements sustained over the next 3 years. We call this approach a Multi-Modal Integrated Therapy for Youth with Bipolar Disorder (MITY-BD, pronounced Mighty-BD).

There's a Rainbow Ahead

We have a lot more work to do, and our research is ongoing, but we know enough now to help you reap the benefits of a system of care that breaks new ground by integrating psychotherapy involving the child and the rest of the family with medication (MITY-BD). What is commonly referred to as "child- and family-focused cognitive-behavioral therapy" (CFF-CBT) is based in part on a model of family-focused therapy with bipolar adults. I have adapted these strategies to meet the unique needs of children with bipolar disorder and added critical elements from interpersonal therapy, and now research is beginning to confirm what I've been seeing in my practice: that children can benefit in the same ways as adults. It is all about finding the right tools for children with bipolar disorder rather than using unmodified tools merely to make do.

Based on a preliminary study I conducted with a small number of patients, when combined with medication, CFF-CBT was shown to decrease the incidence of mania, depression, aggression, psychosis, sleep disturbances, and attention-deficit/hyperactivity disorder (ADHD) and to improve the children's overall functioning. It offers great hope for taming this wild and unpredictable disorder by offering information, encouragement, and tools you can use to move confidently through different stages and situations toward a more positive future for your child and you. It makes you an informed advocate for your child in the outside world—with the healthcare system, schools, and other community institutions that have an impact on your child's well-being and success. Ultimately, psychological treatment plus medication for your child can not only improve your child's quality of life, but also minimize the impact of your child's illness on *your* health (both mental and physical) and that of the rest of your family.

Any therapist who uses cognitive-behavioral therapy, family therapy, or interpersonal therapy will already be familiar with many aspects of the program in this book. Psychotherapy of various types is widely available for children and teens with bipolar disorder, and the most important criterion in choosing a therapist is always the therapist's familiarity with treating these kids. With this book, you can learn how to apply the lessons of our form of treatment on your own and share the information in this book with your child's treatment team.

Because it's easier for children and families to remember, I have boiled down the components of CFF-CBT to seven strategies represented by the acronym RAINBOW. I have infused this entire book with the concepts that make up the RAINBOW approach, and, more important, throughout the book I provide all the information needed to understand bipolar disorder and its relationship with brain function, manage medication, negotiate school situations, persevere through crises, and look after yourself. I'll show you how to apply these principles starting with your child's diagnosis and proceeding through treatment. Chapter 6 in particular breaks down each general strategy into practical tools and techniques you can use to reap the full benefit of your child's treatment and to get your family through every day as unscathed as possible (for now, the display on page 4 shows you what each letter in RAINBOW stands for). But I hope what you'll take from this book more than anything is the ability to apply the concepts and principles of the RAINBOW therapy like they are second nature, translating your new outlook into effective ways to roll with the punches of bipolar disorder in all areas of your unique family's life.

To me, RAINBOW is a neat image for you, your child, and your family to keep in mind, especially when the going gets tough. It symbolizes the happiness and calm that often comes after the storm and serves as a beacon of hope to families in turmoil caused by bipolar disorder. The image of a rainbow is also in keeping with my philosophy that mood variability (represented by the colors of the rainbow) is appropriate in moderation (green versus "ultraviolet" sad moods or "infrared" rages or manic spells, which are more extreme). In my practice, a major goal is to help families incorporate the RAINBOW system into their daily lives so the bipolar child can reach and then stay in the safe middle zone.

The RAINBOW approach helps bipolar children reach that goal by promoting stability both internally and externally. That is, it's called *child- and family-focused therapy* because it targets both the child individually (through medication and individual therapy) and the entire family (through psychoeducation and coping techniques). The underlying premise is that children with bipolar disorder need medication to target the biological source of their mood swings and self-management techniques that will serve them well into adulthood, *but they do even better when their family is doing well too.* RAINBOW keeps the whole family working collaboratively, with an emphasis on positivity. You and your family—and the child, too—will help monitor and manage the child's moods, establish predictable routines and balanced lifestyles, and cultivate supportive friendships for your child and sources of support for you. Your child and the rest of your family will learn to replace negative thinking with positive self-talk and gain experience with the many ways that effective problem solving can keep bipolar disorder from wreaking havoc in your daily lives.

With the **RAINBOW approach,** your family and your child's treatment team help the child stay in the middle of the mood spectrum as much as possible using these strategies (along with medication):

R: *R*outine to encourage a stable schedule

A: *A*ffect (mood) regulation and *A*nger control

I: "*I* can do it"—positive self-talk to build self-esteem

N: *N*o *N*egative thoughts

B: *B*e a good friend (for your child) and lead a *B*alanced lifestyle (for you)

O: *O*ptimal problem solving

W: *W*ays to get support—for the child and the rest of your family

Facing the Challenge Together

"*Everything* is a challenge living with a bipolar child," admits one parent, whether it's "sticking to a constant schedule, always being proactive to prevent the next meltdown, or never knowing what each moment is going to bring." This thought has been echoed by virtually every parent of a bipolar child that I've met. "No matter how diligent you are at understanding the illness and your child's triggers or at preplanning and implementing preventative measures," said one of them, "you have to accept that you will still face the unexpected."

A major goal of the RAINBOW approach is to keep the unexpected to a minimum while acknowledging the reality that it's unlikely to be eliminated altogether. That reality is an example of what I've learned from the hundreds of families like yours who have helped me understand the needs of bipolar children, their parents, and their siblings. The RAINBOW approach emerged not just from my research and clinical experience, but also directly out of the experiences of the families I served. Without their openness and generosity and their unwavering commitment to creating the best possible life for their children, my understanding would be only two-dimensional.

I hope you'll view this book as an extension of the collaboration with families that I've found so fruitful. You and I face the challenges of childhood bipolar disorder together. In this book, I describe in detail how you can work with your own doctor and other caregivers to make the MITY-BD program an effective part of your family's treatment and support system. The nuts and bolts of medication management, therapeutic intervention, and behavior management are only a part of the picture. There's so much more involved. You also need to develop a philosophy and outlook that can get you through the ups and downs, lift you up on the bad days, and help you enjoy the good ones.

That's why I am providing you with a set of principles for coping with the stresses and challenges so eloquently articulated by parents in my practice and throughout this book. I hope these principles will provide a lifeline, as well as a source of inspiration and hope, for coping when times get tough. These principles will show up throughout this book often and in many different forms, and I have summarized them in Appendix A for easy reference.

Look at them often. Mark the page and leave it on your nightstand. Review them before going to bed, and use them to prepare yourself for

Principles for Meeting the Challenges
of Bipolar Disorder

- **Get educated**: Understanding bipolar disorder is one of the first and most important steps you can take to enhance your ability to cope and thrive. Parents invariably report that gaining knowledge about the disorder helps them stay calm, manage their fears, and deal effectively with problems when they arise. As one put it: "I am able to keep my compassion by reading and rereading every bit of information I can about the illness, and by staying in contact with other parents who have similar issues in their homes. The more I know, the less I fear. The less I fear, the more effective I can be in getting treatment for my son and for us."

- **Be realistic**: A diagnosis of bipolar disorder inevitably changes your expectations for your child, yourself, and your family life. You may worry about what kind of future your child will have. Rather than despair about your child's long-term prospects, focus on meeting modest short-term goals like getting through the day without a "meltdown" or having a good outing to the mall. Then celebrate those achievements. Don't expect miracles of your child or yourself, and remember that good things will still happen—find ways to appreciate them when they do.

- **Everything in moderation**: Sometimes parents drive themselves to distraction trying to do everything possible for their child and get everything "right." For instance, keeping a detailed mood chart can take so much time and attention that it gets in the way of your relationship with your child, your spouse, or your other children. Don't let the quest for perfection add to an already stressful situation. You have enough to cope with—do your best with what's important and let some things slide.

- **Be flexible**: If there's any truism of bipolar disorder, it is that unpredictability is the norm, rather than the exception. Your plans can change in an instant and when you least expect it. Being flexible and resilient is not just a good idea, it is a matter of survival for families dealing with bipolar disorder. If flexibility isn't in your nature, it may be a skill you'll have to cultivate.

- **Have fun and learn to play**: Fun doesn't have to go out the window just because your child has bipolar disorder. You both need opportunities to play, relax, and participate in the things that make life worth living. It may seem like a stretch, especially if you've just started down this path, but believe me, you can have fun and find joy in your life if you can get your head above water long enough to look for opportunities.

- **Keep your sense of humor**: It may not seem like there's a lot to laugh about, but you can find plenty of humor if you keep things in perspective. Bipolar kids can be as silly, funny, and clever as other children (sometimes even more so), so enjoy those moments when they amuse, entertain, and delight you. And don't take yourself too seriously. When things go awry despite your best efforts, as they frequently do, recognize the absurdity of it all and remember to take life with a grain of salt. Identify supportive people who can offer strength and stimulate laughter and nurture those friendships.

- **Stay compassionate**: It is a continuing challenge to remain compassionate and loving when your child is at her worst and you're at your wits' end. But your child didn't ask for this disorder nor did she bring it on herself. Try to remember that, as difficult and frustrating as it can be for you, it's even harder for your child. As one parent put it, "What helps me to stay compassionate is insight that I've gained through support groups as to what my son is going through within his mind on a moment-to-moment basis. I can't even imagine how traumatic and difficult it must be to live within himself, hating himself, believing he is stupid and unlovable."

- **Make connections**: You don't have to struggle alone. In fact, isolation is likely to intensify your stress and unhappiness. Build a support network for both your child and yourself. If you find it difficult to identify people you feel comfortable sharing your problems with in your own community, you can connect with thousands of parents facing similar issues online through the Child and Adolescent Bipolar Foundation (CABF) (*www.bpkids.org*), National Alliance on Mental Illness (NAMI) (*www.nami.org*), and similar groups.

whatever tomorrow will bring. Take a few minutes to go over the list to prepare for meetings with doctors, teachers, or other authority figures. Post them on the refrigerator as a reminder for the whole family. Most of all, take them to heart! With these attitudes, you can make such a big difference for your child and the rest of your family.

You Are Your Child's Best Hope

"The thing that helps us stay hopeful is knowing that we have great support (therapist, psychiatrist, school personnel) and that we, as parents, are doing everything we possibly can to help our child."

All parents feel inadequate some of the time, and, given what you are dealing with, you are likely to feel that way more often than most. But if you try your best and keep your expectations modest, patient and consistent parental effort will slowly but surely pay off. When things fall apart, as they occasionally do, remember that you didn't choose this problem, and you have no choice but to keep plugging away. All that you can do is to be the best parent you can be in a difficult situation. So cut yourself some slack, don't work too hard, and don't be too hard on yourself.

The important thing is that you keep your eyes on the horizon. Don't be too discouraged by any setback, whether it lasts a day, a month, or a year. Your child's ultimate outcomes are built slowly over time, and setbacks, regardless of how bad they may be, are almost always temporary. There is always a sunrise after the sunset. What will make a bigger difference than any miracle will be your optimism and the hope that you hold in your heart and convey to your child so that she too can feel it, believe it, and ultimately realize it.

How to Use This Book

You can use this book whether your child has already been diagnosed with bipolar disorder or you're heading in that direction. Some of the strategies, much of the information about bipolar disorder, and all of the principles you'll read about will carry you through to your child's adulthood, but in this book my focus is on children.

The book is divided into three sections, with the chapters moving from the general to the more specific. In Part I, I'll start with an essential foundation of facts and figures that will give you an understanding of the disorder you're dealing with. Part II lays out all the components of the treatment that works and how you can get the best for your child. Part III offers a raft of practical solutions for the daily challenges faced in each domain in which your child spends his days.

You may already know a great deal about bipolar disorder, but I urge you to read Part I anyway, as educating yourself and the other people in your child's life about childhood bipolar disorder is critical to successful treatment and long-term management of the illness. The next few chapters recap some of the latest scientific research, including studies that I've conducted or participated in, and my two decades of clinical experience.

It, and the rest of the book, is also imbued with the wisdom of many parents like you. You'll read about their problems, their hopes, and their creative solutions thanks to the generosity of 200 members of CABF and many other parents from my practice. They, too, are in this with you and me. Together, we'll keep reaching for that rainbow—those beautiful colors arising after the storm!

PART I

The Facts and Fundamentals

KNOWING THE PLAYGROUND

If your child has bipolar disorder, you probably already know a great deal about its symptoms and effects. You've also probably already run the gauntlet of hospitals, doctors, tests, and insurance companies at least once. That experience can turn you into something of an expert overnight!

If you don't think of yourself as an expert but as a frustrated victim, it's time to put on your "positive thinking cap." If you've been dealing with bipolar disorder for some time, you are more of a veteran than you think, with experience to draw from that will allow you to navigate these choppy waters.

Still, chances are you aren't all that confident that you know what's really going on with your child or that you know everything you need to know about the disorder to manage your child's care. You may not even be sure that you have a correct diagnosis or that you have the right doctor, healthcare provider, or support system. You might also be worried about how you're going to pay for care over the long haul, given the state of health insurance today and the potential impact of caring for a bipolar child on your work life (where you may feel you need to look like you're in control when you're really not).

Wherever you are in the process, it will be of help to you, your child, and the rest of your family to understand the "big picture" of bipolar disorder, how it may manifest at different stages in your child's life, and the kind of coexisting problems that can complicate the situation for everyone. This section should give you a very good idea of pediatric bipolar disorder as it is currently understood in the scientific and medical community and should help you make sense of what's happening with your child. It offers a framework to understand the big picture.

Chapters 1–3 are devoted to answering the questions we've found most pressing to parents like you:

- What is bipolar disorder?
- Does it really exist in children?
- What causes it?
- How do you know it is bipolar disorder and not something else?
- Will it get worse or go away in time?
- Will your daughter make it to college and live a normal life?
- Will your son be on medications for the rest of his life?
- Will your child get worse?
- Will he be hospitalized, and when?
- How do you find and choose the best practitioners to help your child?

If you're like most parents today, you've probably done some research on the Internet, and what you've found may have raised more questions than it answered, adding to your anxiety and confusion. My goal in this section is to provide you with accurate, authoritative, state-of-the art information about childhood bipolar disorder, based on my experience as a researcher and pediatric psychiatrist working to develop new approaches to recognize and manage this disorder. I also want to reassure you that, no matter what you've heard, there is hope, and you and your child can make it through! Let me walk through it all with you, as I do with the many families I work with in my practice, and you will see that with the right kind of treatment, support, and encouragement, the future can be bright—even with this difficult and complicated disorder in your lives.

ONE

Yes, Bipolar Disorder Does Occur in Children

Jeremy walks in, wearing a broad smile. He chats garrulously with my staff. He is extremely hyper and starts playing with all the other patients in the waiting area, making rules and bossing them around. Seeing me, he runs up and twists my arm hard as we shake hands. He bursts into laughter as I pull my hand away. His mom, who looks tired and helpless, tells us Jeremy hardly slept the night before. He is chirpy and giggly, talking like a super-express train. He agrees to be videotaped, and my staff goes to get the equipment, but as soon as the camera is set up, his mood changes completely. He starts to direct the filming, then suddenly gets irritable and goes out of control, knocking over the equipment and swearing nonstop.

This is a real example from my clinic. Although somewhat dramatic, stories like these are hardly isolated incidents among bipolar children. Here are a few more examples of things that our patients said or did while in our clinic:

- John (age 10) lifted my research assistants up in his arms; he even attempted to pick up men twice his size and hug strangers, although he would startle and yell if anyone touched him.
- Cindy (age 6) threw herself onto the floor in the hospital corridor and refused to move or get up. She screamed incessantly and turned red in a rage for a half hour before getting blood drawn.
- Jared (age 11) touched everything in sight, talking constantly about things that seemed to have nothing to do with what he was

13

exploring and ricocheting from one topic to the next. "I was thinking that there was this hamster that looked into a mirror and thought there was another hamster and he ran into the mirror!" he said, then laughed hysterically before darting off to another part of my office and telling a story about the time he had "saved" his brother from a dog with "teeth at least a foot long."

- Sylvia (age 9) hid testing materials in our lab in the bottom of a Kleenex box, locked my staff out of the office, threw testing materials away, and jumped up and down in the garbage can.
- Andy (age 7) saw a bird fly against the window of his third-floor playroom and land dazed on the roof below. He climbed out the window and onto the roof in an attempt to help the bird. When his mother retrieved him safely and asked him what he was doing, he responded, "I can fly." His mother reminded him that people can't fly, and he said, "Then God would save me."
- Hannah (age 8) declared, "I'm going to marry you and make you my pretty, pretty princess." She was provocative and overfriendly for a first meeting.
- In the course of 15 minutes during the diagnostic evaluation, Asaad (age 5) went from laughter to yelling and turning red, then broke down crying, unable to articulate his problems given his very young age.
- Joe (age 12) let out a torrent of taunts and criticisms, talking so fast that he was almost incoherent, yelling constantly, rationalizing his anger, and calling his mother a "moron" who had "no brains" as if he were a viciously angry ex-husband.

If your child has received a bipolar diagnosis, or you just suspect that he has the disorder, you may have one of two reactions to these examples. These glimpses of rapid mood swings, irritability, sensitivity to criticism, rapid speech, and difficulty focusing may seem so instantly familiar that you might wonder if someone came into your home and videotaped your child. Maybe your child has behaved in all of these ways at some point. Or you may feel that some of the symptoms match and some don't, that your child is never "that bad," but secretly fear he could get that way. You're not at all sure whether the behaviors depicted above that you *are* seeing in your son or daughter are indicators of bipolar disorder instead of something else entirely.

Even medical professionals have varying reactions to these types of cameos. Either they think these are accurate depictions of childhood bipolar disorder, or they believe that these are difficult behaviors not specific to bipolar disorder, or they dismiss them all as not really bipolar disorder. One parent was often told there was no such "animal" as early-onset or childhood bipolar disorder, and because she was in the mental health field she was accused of "looking for a problem that simply isn't there."

Let me take a minute to clarify how you should view the behaviors portrayed in these very brief stories. The complex emotional turbulence and havoc caused by these children is obvious and dramatic, but parents and professionals should realize that one size does *not* fit all—in other words, no one description captures all the typical bipolar diagnostic symptoms. Your child might have the "classic symptoms," which easily lead to diagnosis, and/or some difficult behaviors, like those described above, which occur more rarely but are definitely associated with the disorder. Because at our clinic we treat hundreds of bipolar children and research their brains and cognitive function, we recognize the wide range of symptoms that can lead to a diagnosis of pediatric bipolar disorder. We think in terms of treating a spectrum of problems related to wiring in the brain that cause dysfunction, rather than just hanging a label on a child based on a diagnosis.

Unfortunately, not everyone recognizes the diagnosis, and there is still a lot of controversy over the label. In this chapter, I hope to clear that up. Make no mistake about it; bipolar disorder does exist in children. The answers to the questions you have about your child's condition aren't always simple or definitive, but they are becoming clearer as brain imaging and clinical research continue to reveal new and useful insights about childhood bipolar disorder each year.

How Is Childhood Bipolar Disorder Defined?

Bipolar disorder is a mood disorder characterized by swings between the opposite and extreme emotional states of mania and depression. The simplest way to put it would be to say that people who have bipolar disorder are sometimes much more "up"—excited, energetic, optimistic, and so forth—than the rest of us and other times much more "down"—that is, sad, dejected, lethargic, and hopeless. But this condition is actually much more complex than that definition implies, and that's why the term "bipolar" is more commonly used today than the older "manic depression"—because it is thought more accurately to reflect the disorder's cyclical nature and the wide variety of symptoms that accompany its two poles (the "bi") of ups and downs. A person suffering from bipolar disorder will not necessarily appear to be energized and happy at one time and visibly sorrowful at another. A person experiencing either mania or depression can seem mainly highly irritable, and the line between the two mood poles isn't always very clear, especially in children.

Differences in the way children manifest bipolar disorder, in fact, are one reason some people doubt that the illness occurs in children at all. Yet we know that it does. Bipolar disorder is said to affect 1–2% of adults worldwide. In one community school survey of older adolescents (aged 14–18 years), some form of bipolar disorder occurred in 1% of them over the course of their lives. It's harder to pin down the incidence of bipolar disorder in children because it is so often misdiagnosed, but, in my opinion, even the rate in teenagers may have been underestimated in the school survey as it was based on interviewing teenagers only, who in most instances deny that anything is ever wrong with them.

When I started my medical training 25 years ago, the idea of bipolar disorder in children was nonexistent. Only adults showing clear signs of mania or elated mood followed by severe depression were recognized as having bipolar disorder. When children with these symptoms came to us for help, we cobbled together several diagnoses to explain their problems and then struggled to understand why they did not respond well to treatment.

The current idea or definition of bipolar disorder in children really started to take shape in the mid-1990s, when new research opened the door to our present understanding. Various researchers looked at the disorder from different angles, each one focusing on a different symptom or dimension as the hallmark of the disease: one focused on irritability, which is a common reason for families to seek treatment for their children; another focused on grandiosity and elated mood; and another stuck to the classic symptoms of mood states that fluctuated from mania to depression similarly to late-adolescent-onset/adult bipolar disorder.

In order to come to a consensus, in 2001, the National Institute of Mental Health (NIMH) convened two Research Roundtables with experts in the field, which produced a general agreement about the main types of bipolar disorder, one based on a narrow definition consisting of the classic symptoms described above and the other a broader definition that encompasses a wide range of symptoms, including severe irritability, "affective storms," mood lability, and severe temper outbursts, falling short of the full set of symptoms or without clearly defined mood cycles. Debate continues between various schools of thought, with some believing that the criteria are being applied too broadly and others feeling that a narrow definition, "the middle cut," leaves out too many children who should be helped.

I, too, erred on the side of caution in diagnosis when I came from

Glossary of Common Terms Associated with Bipolar Disorder

As you get educated about bipolar disorder, it is important to be able to understand some of the common terms you'll encounter in the next few chapters, as well as when you work with doctors, therapists, and others to help your child.

- **Affect**—A pattern of observable behaviors that is the expression of a subjectively experienced feeling state (emotion). Common examples of affect are sadness, elation, and anger. In contrast to mood, which refers to a more pervasive and sustained emotional climate, *affect* refers to a more fluctuating change in emotional "weather." What is considered the normal range of expression of affect varies considerably, both within and among different cultures.
- **Affective storms**—Prolonged and aggressive temper outbursts.
- **Amygdala**—An almond-shaped organ in the lower and inner part of the brain (subcortical structure) that initially receives emotional information and processes it.
- **Anxiety**—Anxiety is a normal response to stress but can become disabling when it is excessive; when it results in unmanageable worries and fears, we call it a disorder.
- **Cognition**—A broad term used to describe brain functioning such as attention (the ability to focus), verbal memory (e.g., the ability to remember what the teacher teaches or says in class), working memory (e.g., the ability to remember shopping lists), executive function (e.g., organization, planning, logical thinking, and problem solving), visual memory (remembering what was seen), visuo–spatial perception (making sense of one's whereabouts, directions to places, etc.), and motor skills (fine-motor skills such as handwriting and gross-motor skills such as kicking a ball). Social cognition has to do with grasping emotions conveyed through facial expressions and social skills.

(cont.)

Glossary of Common Terms *(cont.)*

- **Chronic/ity**—The opposite of acute, meaning that the illness or problems are persistent over an extended period of time. *Chronicity* refers to the state of being chronic, or of long duration.
- **Comorbid**—Two or more disorders occurring at the same time, or coexisting.
- **Depression**—A mood characterized by sadness, diminished pleasure in formerly pleasurable things (*anhedonia*), altered sleep and eating patterns (either more or less than normal), fatigue, agitation and irritability, difficulty concentrating, and a sense of worthlessness; it may include thoughts of suicide.
- **Dysphoria/dysphoric**—A mixed unpleasant mood state that is a combination of irritability, anxiety, and depression.
- **Dysregulation**—Used in this book in relation to mood, where an emotional response is not well modulated or regulated.
- **Dysthymia**—"Flat" mood with little joy, excitement, or happiness that is less severe than depression. It can also include low energy, frequent worry or withdrawal, guilt, irritation, low self-esteem, and sleep and appetite changes.
- **Elated mood**—An abnormally elevated or expansive mood, usually associated with mania, that goes beyond normal childhood happiness and is a qualitative change from what is normal in the child.
- **Excitability**—Being prone to excitement, often associated with elated or manic mood in bipolar disorder.
- **Flights of ideas**—Excessive speech associated with mania in which an individual jumps from topic to topic incessantly, but in this case the topics are related.
- **Hyperactivity**—Behavior that consists of overactive motor activity, usually associated with constant fidgeting, distractibility, impulsivity, and poor concentration or inability to focus.
- **Hypersexuality**—In bipolar children, this symptom manifests in acting flirtatious beyond their years and disinhibited, excessively looking at pornographic pictures or constantly visiting websites with sexual material, touching the private areas of adults or other youth (including teachers, parents, siblings, and acquaintances), and using explicit sexual language.
- **Hypomania**—A mild to moderate level of symptoms of elated mood, irritability, high energy, flights of ideas, pressured speech, and poor sleep. The only difference between manic and hypomanic symptoms is that young people with the latter do not require hospitalization and can function without major turbulence.

- **Impulsivity**—An inclination to act without thinking about the consequences. An impulsive child may have trouble waiting for his or her turn, interrupt or blurt out answers, or take risks.
- **Irritability**—A state of being easily angered or aggressive, which can show up in bipolar children as hostility or sarcasm, out-of-proportion responses to events, or outright raging.
- **Lability**—Abnormal variability in affect with repeated, rapid, and abrupt shifts in affective expressions.
- **Mood**—A pervasive and sustained emotion that colors one's perception of the world. Common examples of mood include depression, elation, anger, and anxiety.
- **Mixed mood**—An emotional state characterized by simultaneous symptoms of mania and depression.
- **Oppositionality**—Refusal to comply with ordinary requests or willful defiance of authority.
- **Prefrontal cortex**—A region in the brain's frontal lobe. It has many parts to it and acts as a higher center for modulating affect as well as controlling all cognitive functions.
- **Pressured speech**—Rapid, nonstop, driven talking that may come out so fast as to be unintelligible, like a horrendous flow of speech being forced out through a narrow hole.
- **Psychosis**—Loss of contact with reality in which there is qualitative change; an individual hears things (auditory hallucinations) or sees things (visual hallucinations) that are not there, believes in things that are not true (i.e., fixed false beliefs, or delusions, particularly paranoid or grandiose delusions in bipolar disorder), and communicates in garbled, incoherent speech (thought disorder; particularly flights of ideas in bipolar disorder).
- **Reactivity**—An emotional response to an outside event or externally or internally generated perceptions that are unusually strong or sudden.
- **Temperament**—A basic cluster of biological characteristics that a person is born with such as affect regulation, reactivity, sleep patterns, sociability, flexibility, and how easy it is to soothe the child. Difficult temperament is often associated with bipolar disorder.

Australia to the United States in late 1990s. I used to diagnose what we now think of as childhood bipolar disorder as attention-deficit/hyperactivity disorder (ADHD) (as children with bipolar disorder are hyperactive and distractible) + oppositional defiant disorder (ODD) (as they are irritable and difficult but short of conduct problems) + major depression (as they had mixed depressive symptoms). This diagnosis still did not address these children's elated mood, grandiosity, excitability and exuberance, creative and excessive productivity, flights of ideas and pressured speech, sleep difficulties, or hypersexuality. We could not control their emotional dysregulation. Like most of my colleagues, I treated these children with stimulants or antidepressants, with poor results. It was like the fable of the blind men trying to describe an elephant—we defined the problem based on the part we were touching at the time.

I spent significant amounts of time investigating the syndrome to understand it better. I began to attract patients from all over the country and abroad, and in the course of treating them, a pattern emerged. I saw that the mood fluctuations weren't just a matter of temperament. They worsened with age. In addition, the symptoms and cycles didn't behave exactly like bipolar disorder in adults (see the box below). Two big things convinced me that this was a distinct disorder that manifested itself in children uniquely: (1) treating it as simply ADHD, depression, or a combination of the two did not do the trick; it was much more complicated than any of these other conditions; and (2) treating it like adult bipolar disorder seemed to help these children, although there were some important differences owing to brain development and their youth when symptoms began.

Bipolar disorder can be difficult to diagnose (and treat) in children because it differs from the same disorder in adults in these ways:

- Children may experience mixed episodes (i.e., the symptoms of mania and depression coexist at the same time or alternate much more rapidly between mania and depression than in adults).
- Children are more irritable. While this is not the defining feature, it is very common.
- Coexisting ADHD-like symptoms. As hyperactivity, impulsivity, and inattention are common in both bipolar disorder and ADHD, it is hard to know if they are overlapping symptoms or two disorders occurring together.
- Rapid cycling, in which the child yo-yos between high and low moods within a single day.
- Chronic symptoms with poor rates of remission unless the child is receiving treatment.

I felt compelled to do something to help bipolar children who desperately need attention for this poorly understood and ill-treated disorder. Although we don't yet fully understand the disorder or its causes, we must start treating it while our understanding of the brain and nervous system continues to evolve. Rather than being submerged in debate, we must apply these scientific findings to making a difference *now* for kids in the real world and not keep them waiting! I believe it is better to embrace an imperfect label and do what's right by treating these suffering kids.

Considering how your child is undoubtedly struggling, I'm sure you'll agree. So let's take time right now to clear up a myth that all too often stands in the way of getting help for bipolar children: that you, rather than a biological illness, are to blame for your child's problems. You are a blessing that your child can count on, not a curse that caused the disorder.

Is Your Child Just Acting Out in Response to Poor Parenting?

Whether your child is just "acting out" rather than suffering from an illness is a question that can be answered only through a thorough diagnostic evaluation of the sort described in Chapter 2. But if your child does meet the diagnostic criteria, I can tell you without reservation that *you are not to blame for your child's behavior or any other aspect of the illness.* We know that bipolar disorder is a biologically based illness that tends to run in families; it is not caused by parenting style or any other environmental influences. If you are too reactive and there is emotional friction in the family, it is not healthy for you or anybody, including your bipolar child. It does not mean you are causing the disorder, but you may be fueling the fire inadvertently. So, slowing down, thinking with clarity, and monitoring oneself in the process is a very good thing to do. Unfortunately, the behavior of a bipolar child can be so hard to manage that you may very well feel like a terrible parent, and you may still fall prey to the sorts of fault-finding described in the box on pages 22–23. Education—of yourself and others—is the best antidote. A good place to start is with an understanding of the biological basis of bipolar disorder.

Scientists have yet to identify a specific cause for bipolar disorder, and there is no one test that can be performed to confirm or rule out the disorder; however, studies point to a number of genetic and physiological factors that may play a role in the onset of the disorder and some psycho-

Dispelling the "Bad Parenting" Myth

"I blamed myself for my son's behavior for years before I sought help of any kind. He was my first child and all my friends had their first kids and none of their kids behaved like my son. My parents and my in-laws also made me feel like I was a bad parent when he was young, giving me all kinds of advice on how to discipline him."

"One friend told me that my son simply needed more exercise, specifically swimming. I have endured terrible glares and pointed comments from strangers in stores about my kids' behavior. My least favorite, though, is when someone tries to convince me that BP isn't real, or that the medications my children are taking are actually the cause of their behaviors!"

Parents of bipolar children are often unfairly criticized for their child's problem, as if bad parenting were to blame for bipolar disorder and its many symptoms. It is the height of emotional abuse of parents to say this! Where does this blame and hostility come from? The problem is often grounded in cultural stereotypes and ignorance about childhood bipolar disorder. The rigid and uninformed views of spouses, relatives, neighbors, teachers, and even some doctors can get in the way. This criticism is often subtle or indirect and can manifest in several ways:

- Fathers will sometimes accuse mothers of imagining or exaggerating the child's symptoms (e.g., "Johnny is fine around me; he's perfectly normal"). Of course, because the father is around less often, he witnesses less misbehavior. Dad also usually wields more authority in the home, so the bipolar child may be on her best behavior when he is around. More important, these children may be more intimate with their mother and feel freer to express their anger to her. Sometimes it's the father who is accused of being a pushover for an "out-of-control" child, but, more often than not, it's Mom who bears the brunt of criticism.
- Grandparents or in-laws accuse the parents of creating a "monster" by being too permissive. As previous generations viewed mothers as playing the central role in parenting (I am afraid this role actually has not changed much), the child's misbehavior is seen as a disciplining failure on the mother's part.
- Even doctors, particularly "old-schoolers" who might not be up on the latest research, can be quick to criticize parents for imagining things or jumping to conclusions, especially if they don't believe that bipolar

disorder exists in children. This is magnified because bipolar children are more likely to act completely normal in the doctor's office. One parent was told by a doctor that "we were not disciplining our son, that we needed to make it known to him that we were the parents, that he had to mind us, and that if he had to sit in his room day after day to understand this concept, then that is what we needed to do." Meanwhile, symptoms continue unabated, and the parents, who may have been praised for raising so-called "normal" children, lose their self-confidence. When the medication works and children respond, it almost seems like a miracle. Suddenly one's parenting skills appear quite adequate, even profound! Again and again, I see parents vindicated when their child finally gets the right diagnosis and treatment.

- In extreme cases, parents may be accused by doctors, teachers, or other professionals of sexual abuse, particularly if they happen to witness the hypersexuality that is one of the common clinical features of bipolar disorder. Of course, sexual abuse is not unheard of these days, but a doctor who jumps to this conclusion and blames an innocent parent may cause more harm to the child and family than the illness itself.

- In another all-too-common scenario, parents (usually a mother) may be accused of Munchausen syndrome (i.e., making up an illness in their child to elicit attention or sympathy for themselves). A doctor may think the mother has exaggerated her child's symptoms—including extreme destruction and rage attacks during manic episodes— because the child behaves like a "sweet little angel" in the office. The unintended result is litigation, heartbreak, and, of course, more symptoms. How do you save yourself from such accusations? Instead of reciting the diagnostic symptoms in an effort to make it easy for the doctor, give concrete examples of what went wrong. For example, I will ask: "Describe three to five very difficult times with your child or talk about the three situations that worried you the most." This kind of information gives the clinician a good feel for how the illness waxes and wanes or unfolded in the first place and easily identifies the real cases.

If these injustices are still happening to your child and family, try to find a professional who really understands bipolar disorder and can offer the correct diagnosis. The self-doubt, guilt, and shame others might try to heap on you can only hurt and prevent you and your child from getting help. You need to step out from under that cloud and find supportive and knowledgeable doctors who can help. See Chapter 3 for more insight on choosing the right doctor and team.

logical and social factors that can determine its severity and the child's (and family's) ability to cope. In the future, further studies of these "markers" or risk factors may eventually lead to improvements in the prevention, diagnosis, and treatment of bipolar disorder in children and adults.

Did My Child Inherit This Illness?

There is growing evidence that a predisposition toward bipolar disorder is an inherited trait. Both top-down and bottom-up studies show a strong pattern of family inheritance. In top-down studies, researchers start with members of the older generation with the disorder and track signs of the disorder in these adults' children. Bottom-up studies identify bipolar disorder in children and then look for signs of it in their adult relatives.

One study based on detailed interviews with parents of outpatient children or adolescents with type I bipolar disorder (where children experience full-blown mania and depression versus a "lower grade" of mania known as hypomania in addition to depression; see Chapter 2 for more on the subtypes of bipolar disorder) found that roughly 80% of these children had at least one parent diagnosed with a mood disorder. Several studies have shown a strong link between early age of onset and risk of bipolar disorder among first-degree relatives as compared to relatives of youth with schizophrenia, unipolar major depressive disorder, and normal controls. Further, earlier onset of bipolar disorder is associated with greater odds of having bipolar disorder in the family. Relatives of adolescents with variable symptoms also have increased family history of bipolar disorder, comparable to those with the full syndrome. Relatives of children with ADHD and bipolar disorder are five times more likely to have bipolar disorder than relatives of children who only have ADHD. This statistic makes the scientist in me speculate about whether ADHD and bipolar disorder are somehow related and whether ADHD is symptomatic of bipolar tendencies, as bipolar children often are identified as having ADHD before full-blown bipolar disorder emerges. We don't know if these children get worse because of wrong or harmful stimulant medications or because they are predisposed to develop bipolar disorder anyway.

The genetics of bipolar disorder raises two important issues for families. First, parents frequently feel guilty about "giving" the disorder to their child, even when they might not be affected themselves. Guilt can interfere with effectively parenting a bipolar child and can lead to marital discord and other family conflict. Often, I hear mothers (or occasionally fathers) refer to an undiagnosed partner as having passed along the symptoms. In the heat of the moment, people will say things like "the apple doesn't fall far from the tree." Even when it's true, it is wielded as a negative judgment toward the affected parent, which is particularly common if the parents are divorced. It may, in fact, be true that you passed along the predisposition to bipolar disorder, but it's not as if you did this intentionally or as if there were anything you could have done to prevent it. What's important to know is that there is plenty you can do to make it better for your child.

Second, if you happen to be affected by the disorder and are unaware of it, you are as much a victim as your child. Mood swings can be exhausting even if you've found ways to compensate and prevent them from interfering in your life. Coping with a mood disorder yourself along with trying to manage your child's mood disorder can multiply the amount of stress you and your child experience. For example, among families with a bipolar child, our laboratory and others have reported greater amounts of problematic and conflictual family functioning when one or both parents were also diagnosed with a mood disorder. I hope, therefore, that you and your child's other parent will consider whether you may need help for mood symptoms of your own, whether the cause is bipolar disorder, depression, or stress. The fact that parents with undiagnosed mood problems can inadvertently reinforce certain symptoms in a bipolar child means that getting that help is another way you can help your son or daughter. Remember that a large percentage of parents do not have a bipolar disorder!

The bottom line is that *you are not to blame.* Not every at-risk child develops the disorder, so don't beat yourself up. Bipolar disorder often goes unrecognized in a family—everyone thinks that Uncle George is just moody or unlucky or both. In fact, after you learn about the symptoms, you may even discover that someone in the family may have been affected by the disorder and has not received the help he or she needs either. Now is the chance for that individual to obtain the information, medication, and support he or she needs, so no one has to suffer anymore.

Was My Child Born Different?

New imaging techniques are allowing scientists to look at the structure and functioning of the brain to see how they may differ in individuals with bipolar disorder. Complicating factors such as coexisting conditions, the phase of the illness the person is in during testing (e.g., depressed, manic, hypomanic, euthymic), and the presence of multiple medications make it difficult to make definitive statements about brain function. Over the past three decades, there have been several interesting studies that suggest that the brains of children with bipolar disorder may be structurally and functionally different in ways related to their thinking, emotions, perceptions of other people, and control over their behavior.

Structural studies showed a smaller amygdala (an almond-sized organ at the bottom of the brain that receives and processes emotions first) in these children. We also are beginning to understand that the prefrontal lobe, which functions as the "the CEO of the brain," does not operate effectively in children with bipolar disorder in the same way as in children who don't have the disorder. As a result, it does not effectively modulate the excessively active amygdala, which receives and processes emotions. Top-down regulation, therefore, seems to be impaired, especially when the bipolar child is provoked by negative experiences. In one of our studies, showing angry faces to bipolar kids elicited an unusually strong emotional reaction, suggesting that these children may not interpret facial cues accurately compared to nonbipolar children. Similarly, we showed that prefrontal activity was inefficient when exposed to negative words like "jerk" and "stupid." Even the part of the prefrontal cortex that is useful in maintaining attention and helps problem-solve (the dorsolateral part of the prefrontal cortex) shuts down in response to negative emotions. Whether these variations are the cause of bipolar disorder or the effect of the illness on the developing brain is still unclear and requires further study, but the results certainly tell us that emotions are poorly regulated in these children, leading to reactivity, excessive sensitivity to criticism, and extreme responses to stress.

We and several other experts have unanimously shown that brain function in bipolar children is compromised in ways that directly impact learning. Regardless of how smart they are, bipolar children have problems with attention, memory for heard/spoken information (called verbal memory), memory for holding small amounts of information like shopping lists or math facts to complete task at hand (called working memory), and difficulty with problem solving, transitioning organization, and planning ahead (otherwise known as the "executive functions"). Addressing mood alone may not help fix these problems, and active educational interventions may be needed. I will provide more information on what to do about learning problems associated with bipolar disorder in Chapter 9.

How We Know It's Biology and Not You

- As many as three quarters of all kids and teens with bipolar disorder may have inherited it from a parent.
- There's evidence of a stronger genetic link in bipolar disorder than in schizophrenia and other mental illnesses that appear in young people.
- We find a family connection when we look both ways—at the parents of bipolar kids and at the children of bipolar adults.
- There are structural differences in the brains of bipolar children, such as a smaller amygdala.
- Children with bipolar disorder have problems with brain function in areas such as the prefrontal cortex and amygdala that affect emotion regulation, thinking, and learning ability.

Does This Mean Parenting Plays No Role?

Parenting *does* play a role in your child's well-being, though nothing you do or have done as a parent can predispose your child to having bipolar disorder. In other words, what goes on at home didn't give your child bipolar disorder, but it can certainly influence how well your child (and your family) weathers the mood storms. While the exact mechanism is unknown, psychosocial factors—the psychological makeup of parents, family dynamics, and other socializing influences—play a role in childhood bipolar disorder. A study by Dr. Barbara Geller and her colleagues reported that more than half of children and teenagers diagnosed with bipolar disorder had difficulty getting along with friends and were teased by other children. They also had poor relationships with siblings and conflict with their parents. This is understandable, given their tendency to be intense, jealous, and intrusive with siblings and argumentative with parents. It is sad, but it appears that a high degree of hostility and lower levels of warmth with children compromised negotiation skills and limited agreement between parents on how to raise and discipline these children. It is quite understandable how bipolar kids push you to your limit till you feel guilty about how rageful or desperate you can feel at times. As the frustration builds up, everyone suffers: "I did not have another child because of the intensity of caring for her," said one parent. "It alters plans, schedules, maximizes doctor's appointments and meetings, disrupts careers, etc. I have seen it destroy and negatively impact both siblings and marriages." Another mother found that the disorder negatively influenced her own behavior in a number of ways: "Sometimes I say things that I know don't help him or I get on his case for not helping out around the house at all. I have a lot of guilt, too, for letting him get away with things that I would never let his brothers get away with." It's easy to see how relationships can deteriorate under the strain of living with a bipolar child, which reinforces the need to involve the whole family in treatment and management of childhood bipolar disorder.

Does the stress of growing up in a home with a bipolar parent predispose a child to develop the disorder? Certainly such children are not only genetically at risk, but also more likely to be exposed to negative life events than children and adolescents of nonbipolar parents. Few studies, however, have evaluated the effects of these stresses on the onset and maintenance of childhood bipolar disorder. We found high rates of conflict and quarrels between parents and children with bipolar disorder. A number of factors compound this conflict, as informed by our research, such as an earlier age of illness onset, a coexisting ADHD diagnosis in the child, parental mood disorder, and parents being single or divorced. All of these factors add significantly to the stress level of these parents and contribute to stressful parent–child relationships.

How Do We Know It's Really Bipolar Disorder?

In this chapter, I've summed up how we know that bipolar disorder exists in children—it's a distinct disorder, and it *is* bipolar disorder even though it may look like something else and it may *not* look the way bipolar disorder typically looks in adults. Understanding that this is a real illness and it has a name, as well as that it's biologically and genetically based and not just a behavior pattern caused by parents, shuts the door on fruitless debates that simply delay the treatment your child needs. In the next chapter, I'll talk more about how bipolar disorder is diagnosed, its common symptoms, and the many related issues that can make it challenging—but possible—to treat long term.

TWO

Does My Child
Really Have Bipolar Disorder?

At times all children exhibit some of the same behaviors as the bipolar child—they can be highly active, imaginative, boastful, and sensitive to criticism. Any child will "act out" once in a while, become giddy, play the clown, or become inexplicably irritable. But if your child has received a diagnosis of bipolar disorder or is having more than an occasional meltdown, you know your child's behavior isn't just like everyone else's.

Experienced clinicians define what is "abnormal" by comparing the severity and persistence of a child's symptoms to the average or "norm," given the child's age and stage of development as well as the situation or setting in which the behavior occurs. We look for a specific cluster of classic symptoms: extremely elated giddy behavior, extreme irritability with rages, risk taking, and/or grandiose statements. For example, a bipolar adult in the throes of mania might say, "I can run the world," while a bipolar child might say, "I can run the school." These children are smart enough to know that this is illogical. That kind of calculated hyperbole illustrates the difference between abnormal behavior and the occasional silly statements that all kids make.

What Does Bipolar Disorder Look Like?

Here are the signs of pediatric bipolar disorder that clinicians typically look for, based on the *Diagnostic and Statistical Manual of Mental Disorders* (DSM), the American Psychiatric Association's diagnostic "bible," which reflects the consensus of mental health professionals working in this field today:

- **_Elated mood_** often shows up as being excitable, silly, giddy, and feeling invincible and "overwhelmed," combined with laughing fits and excessive joking. For example, your child rolls on the floor laughing or appears "over the top." "It is overwhelming," said one child. "I feel like jumping on the bed nonstop."

- **_Irritable mood_** shows up as being easily irritated and aggressive, raging, throwing things, slamming doors, having difficulty transitioning from one activity to another, being hostile or sarcastic, kicking, screaming, and showing intense and inconsolable responses out of proportion to the situation. The children may apologize to their parents later: "I said, 'No, no, no,' to my brain, but it can't stop being mad." Parents often say, "we are walking on eggshells" waiting for an outburst. One parent likened it to living "in a war zone—I never know when new battles will erupt or fighting needs to be stopped. We live in an almost constant state of crisis." One child in our clinic threw his parent's coat in the toilet and their food in the garbage. His mother remarked that "even the family dog is hiding from him; that is usually when I know he is in a bad cycle."

- **_Inflated self-esteem and grandiosity_** are characterized by unsupported statements such as "I am the best baseball player in America"; "I will teach the coach how to swim; he has no clue"; "I am absolutely sure I will get an Oscar before I'm 35"; "I am going to make millions through e-trading"; "I do not need to go to school"; "I am the queen of the universe. You are beneath me"; "This disease will be named after me after I die at 30. I just know it." As with adults, psychosis is often seen in the manic phase. Delusions of grandeur can be separated from bragging if the age-appropriate reality check is absent and the child acts on the delusions. Sometimes a bossy/grandiose sense of self (talking and acting like he or she knows everything and can do anything) comes from inflated self-esteem or grandiosity short of delusions. Some people think the child is just narcissistic; although it may look that way, this behavior appears only in a manic phase. At the same time, it is important to know that these children may also have underlying insecurities and low self-esteem that make them narcissistic in addition to the waxing and waning sense of grandiosity. I am not trying to make it complicated, but the personality is affected by chronic illness, and there can be symptoms on top of the illness.

• **Decreased need for sleep** is illustrated by parents' descriptions of their children playing, singing, or watching television into the early morning, refusing to go to bed, and still not feeling tired in the morning. Children often describe their subjective experience as feeling like the Energizer bunny. Young children are often seen playing in their room late at night. They jump out of bed before the crack of dawn. Conversely, they may exhibit this symptom infrequently or not at all—they may go to sleep quite late or take medications that make them groggy and consequently have difficulty getting out of bed in the morning.

• **Pressure to keep talking and flights of ideas** are often illustrated by statements like "My mind is like a Ferrari; a million thoughts are racing. I can't stop it"; "No stoppers"; "My mind is like a ship with too many passengers, all talking." A mother might say to me: "Listen to his rambling, Doctor. Does it make sense?" Parents describe these children as constantly talking, never letting others have a say, domineering, and continually seeking attention by talking excessively or being unable to stop entertaining at home or school. Some children even invent their own language, switching back and forth between invented words.

• **Constant goal-directed activity** is illustrated by continually fiddling and making a mess at home. When parents confront the mess or spills, the children become defensive, denying that they are responsible. In our experience, parents report this as "lying." It takes some effort to piece together the history of these "frenzied episodes." One child described himself as going through "crazy maniacal spells." Another child reported: "I ran for class president and I lost, but I'm fund raising to organize a rock concert. There is a lot to do. Let's get started." Parents may describe constant goal-directed behavior such as feeding the dog, playing chess, doing art, and fighting with siblings all in 1 hour.

• **Excessive pleasurable activities (hypersexuality), poor judgment, and risk taking:** Youngsters may call sex lines; suddenly start dressing inappropriately; get on sexually oriented chat lines; masturbate excessively; cut, hoard, or carry pornographic pictures; simulate sexual activity with animals; use their parents' credit cards to order sex items by mail; or pressure parents to buy expensive dresses or other items. Sometimes, they even involve parents—for instance, wearing their mother's underwear, calling her "Mr. Fuck," hugging her from behind in an awkward manner, or touching her breasts. When this occurs, sexual abuse is often suspected, but, according to an ongoing study, only a small fraction of bipolar children (1.1%) have a history of sexual abuse or overstimulation, while 43%

exhibited hypersexuality. This data supports the idea that this behavior is a critical symptom in bipolar disorder. Similarly, these children may exhibit poor judgment about what they can and cannot do or take more extreme physical risks than other children. Parents report that, when in the grips of an extreme mood swing, their bipolar children can be dangerously impulsive and destructive, for instance, trying to jump out of an upstairs window or moving vehicle, cutting up clothing, or destroying furniture.

• *Features of depression* are often described in age-specific terms. Children may report feeling crabby, whine excessively, cry for no reason, look unhappy, spend hours in a dark room, change moods rapidly from irritable to tearful, engage in skin pinching and self-scratching at a young age, or complain of somatic symptoms, such as stomachaches and headaches. These children often develop intense sensitivity to rejection from years of negative response from others because of their prickly and cyclic behavior.

Common Symptoms of Bipolar Disorder in Children

- Does your child become overly excited, giddy, and silly in a way that seems "over the top" compared to other kids and for the situation?
- Does your child get highly irritated and out of control, seeming unable to control aggravation and anger that are out of proportion to the circumstances?
- Does your child make grandiose claims of superiority, beyond the realm of typical childish bragging, and think and act as if he or she "knows it all" or is superior to others?
- Does your child have trouble going to sleep or staying asleep, with little sign of exhaustion due to sleep deprivation?
- Does your child talk nonstop and complain of not being to halt the thoughts flooding his or her mind?
- Does your child get lost in project after project, never seeming to tire of planning and pursuing these plans?
- Does your child display signs of "hypersexuality," that is, a precocious knowledge of or interest in private parts, self-stimulation, or sexual language?
- Does your child take risks other kids don't take, seeming unconfined by the boundaries of common sense?
- Does your child have bouts with sadness, crying, whining, and dejection for no apparent reason?

If Your Child Doesn't Have the Most Common Symptoms, Does It Mean He or She Doesn't Have Bipolar Disorder?

Diagnosis is more an art than a science. In the case of a complicated illness like bipolar disorder, it is impossible to make a diagnosis based on a simple checklist. Your child may have all or just some of the typical symptoms or have others not usually included in the DSM criteria. For example, some children just exhibit extreme irritability with few other symptoms; these children may have issues similar to children who have more classic bipolar disorder, but fall into a broad spectrum known as "atypical bipolar disorder." In general, however, if your child shows the following signs, there is a **significant chance** he has bipolar disorder:

- Mood is the central problem, with the child having mania or mania mixed with depression for more than 4 days in a row at a time.
- The child cycles rapidly from being excitable, silly, and giggly to being irritable or depressed, sulky, withdrawn, and deeply sad.
- Psychotic symptoms, such as seeing or hearing things, may or may not be present and are not necessary to make the diagnosis.

- *Threats of suicide:* Even very young bipolar children and preteens may report suicidal behavior, stating a desire to hang or choke themselves. This usually represents desperate attempts to regulate or escape from the intense mood swings. Suicidal behavior is reported to be as high as 25% in childhood bipolar disorder. Suicide attempts in young children may often be mistaken as risk-taking behavior or accidents, such as running in front of a moving car, jumping out of a moving car, or jumping from a tree house.

- *Psychosis* may show up as auditory or visual hallucinations, usually in addition to the mood-based delusions described earlier. What may start out as a rapid flight of ideas could become a garbled, incoherent torrent of words. Depending on the reporting method, psychosis may be present in from 17 to 60% of bipolar patients. During psychotic depressive episodes, delusions of doom, disaster, and nihilism are common. For example, one child drew pictures of a black ghost trying to take over the world.

All these symptoms are seldom present in one child and certainly not at one time. **Generally speaking, cyclical changes in mood, from very** happy to very sad with episodes of irritability, anxiety, and extreme "reactivity," are most commonly seen in children with bipolar disorder. Significant ongoing behavior problems that affect relationships and functioning, such as extreme rebelliousness, delusional thinking, paranoia, academic failure, or threats of suicide or violence, are also very common in kids with bipolar disorder.

How Do Doctors Diagnose Bipolar Disorder?

Bipolar disorder is not a "one-size-fits-all" condition. It can look quite different in different children and at different times. The frequency, depth, and duration of moods can vary a great deal from child to child. It can even change as your child goes through different stages of development.

Does it really matter what kind of bipolar disorder your child has? After all, your child is still suffering. However, it may matter a great deal if your child's symptoms do not fit a "typical" pattern and, as a result, you have trouble getting a correct diagnosis or treatment. If the subtypes discussed below prove anything, it is that bipolar disorder is a complex and confounding condition in children that requires a thorough evaluation to identify and treat. To my way of thinking, it also demonstrates that it is time to stop debating whether bipolar disorder exists in children and teach doctors how to screen properly for this difficult disease. Let's bring some compassion and common sense to the situation.

In the DSM-IV, the American Psychiatric Association has identified the following main subtypes of childhood bipolar disorder:

• **Bipolar I:** This label is used to describe children who have had at least one manic or "mixed" episode (characteristics of both mania—the first seven symptoms described above—and depression occurring nearly every day for at least a 1-week period). These children have periods of extreme euphoria or irritability and rages alternating with marked periods of depression; however, children who have not shown any signs of depression can still be diagnosed with bipolar I disorder; all that is required is mania.

"Rapid cycling" can occur in children diagnosed with bipolar I, which means that the child's mood changes from one extreme to the other at least four times per year. "Ultrarapid cycling" or "ultrafine cycling" differs from what is described in the DSM and involves rapid, pendulum-like mood swings occurring any time from every 2 days to every hour.

- **Bipolar II:** This diagnosis is applied to children who experience periods of major depression and at least some manic symptoms, such as grandiosity, decreased need for sleep, pressured speech, flights of ideas, etc. Here, you'll see a qualitative change in behavior, with your child exhibiting some "hypomania," meaning that your child will be somewhat manic but remain functional and the symptoms will not last for more than 4 days in a row. Mixed episodes and rapid cycling can occur here as well.

- **Cyclothymia:** These children may alternate between symptoms of hypomania and symptoms of low-grade depression, but not exhibit full-blown depression or mania. When we see a child whose moods cycle but who can still function, we think of this diagnosis as long as the depression is relatively less severe.

- **Bipolar not otherwise specified (NOS):** Children who do not meet all the preceding criteria in either the pattern or duration of symptoms but have a mood disturbance and are functionally impaired will often be labeled bipolar NOS. These include children who demonstrate severe irritability and chronic and continuous presence of symptoms with no episodic changes. They may or may not experience elated mood or grandiosity. Although these children have fewer symptoms or can be less severe, they are still very ill, yet do not fit into a clear symptom pattern.

- **Bipolar I:** Full-blown mania or mixed episodes, which may or may not alternate with depression.
- **Bipolar II:** Major depression with lower-grade mania (hypomania), with the ability to function without needing hospitalization.
- **Cyclothymia:** Cycling between low-grade mania and low-grade depression with basic functioning preserved.
- **Bipolar NOS:** Mood problems that fall short of the criteria for bipolar I and II in terms of pattern or duration of symptoms but may vary from mild to extremely severe. This is the most common variant of childhood bipolar disorder.

What Else Could Be Affecting My Child?

Some popular books on the subject depict the most extreme symptoms of bipolar disorder, such as psychosis, sexual behavior, threats of suicide, or violence, in order to build empathy for these suffering individuals. Scientists correctly try to focus on the common core symptoms, such as mood swings, irritability, anxiety, and reactivity, not wanting to be swayed by these seemingly exaggerated examples. Unfortunately, extreme symptoms like these occur at varying rates in a significant number of bipolar children. Sometimes, these symptoms are the result of other conditions that occur alongside bipolar disorder and may not be fully accounted for by the bipolar diagnosis.

More often than not, children and adolescents with bipolar disorder have at least one other psychiatric disorder at the same time—these are referred to as "comorbid" conditions and typically include ADHD, oppositional defiant disorder (ODD), conduct disorder (CD), anxiety disorders, and, more commonly in adolescents, substance abuse disorders.

There is little agreement among researchers as to how common these comorbid disorders are, as estimates vary widely according to the age of the child, the child's background, the research methodology, and the diagnostic criteria used. Rates for comorbid disorders range widely between 10 and 75% for ADHD; 45 and 75% for ODD; 5 and 40% for CD; 12 and 60% for anxiety disorders; and 0 and 40% for substance abuse disorders.

Types of comorbid conditions vary significantly based on the age of the child. Bipolar children tend to have higher rates of ADHD than adolescents, while the latter have higher rates of substance abuse—in fact, the risk of substance abuse was around 9 times higher in adolescent-onset bipolar disorder than in pediatric bipolar disorder. Bipolar disorder can be associated with autism spectrum disorders, also known as pervasive developmental disorders (PDD), in around 10% of cases. Asperger syndrome is a variant of this disorder where children present with limited empathy and social skills but generally tend to have good language skills.

How to Distinguish Bipolar Disorder from Other Conditions

The symptoms of bipolar disorder and other psychiatric disorders frequently overlap, so it can be difficult to differentiate bipolar disorder from these conditions, particularly ADHD. Unfortunately, misdiagnosis can have serious consequences. For instance, placing a bipolar child on a stimulant used to treat ADHD can worsen manic symptoms! So, it's important to know how to tell bipolar disorder and other syndromes apart and manage them properly, whether they coexist with bipolar disorder or not. Failure to diagnose and treat a comorbid condition can also affect your child's progress, making it difficult to tell whether a particular treatment program is working as expected.

Attention-Deficit/Hyperactivity Disorder (ADHD)

ADHD is a lifelong disorder that generally appears in childhood and remains constant over time. It is difficult to get a clear diagnosis of bipolar disorder as symptoms such as inattention, hyperactivity, and impulsivity overlap with ADHD. Doctors typically must rely on parents' reports to identify whether these symptoms are cyclical or not. Irritability that is seen in bipolar disorder and ADHD is also present in ODD and depression, further complicating diagnosis.

For example, a child named Tom came to our clinic with severe rages, increased energy, decreased sleep, and symptoms of depression. The depressive symptoms came and went, but he had always been hyperactive. Tom received treatment for ADHD from age 5 to 7 years. Stimulant medication really helped. His parents could not remember ever seeing aggression or mood fluctuations until he turned 7. Suddenly, the clinical picture became more complicated. Symptoms became cyclical, with ADHD and low-grade mood symptoms alternating with full-blown bipolar episodes. Although it seemed chronic, there were brief periods of 4 days to 2 weeks of "relative calm."

We have shown in our research that bipolar disorder is associated

---

ADHD and Bipolar Disorder

ADHD only	Shared symptoms	Bipolar only
Early onset	Inattention	Fluctuating symptoms, but also often chronic
Constant symptoms	Impulsivity	
	Irritability	Grandiosity
		Elation
		Hypersexuality
		Flights of ideas
		Decreased need for sleep

with cognitive problems combined with poor attention regardless of ADHD, which are likely to remain even after you treat mood symptoms. If a child is diagnosed with both disorders, we recommend treating bipolar disorder as the primary disorder (regardless of ADHD) and addressing the symptoms of ADHD secondarily if they still exist. That way, you are not likely to produce mania by giving stimulants. Stimulants worsen manic symptoms in a portion of bipolar kids, but we don't know which children are vulnerable in this way and which ones are not. Thus, doctors must approach the treatment of bipolar disorder combined with ADHD very carefully.

Clinicians generally believe that there are five key symptoms that differentiate bipolar disorder from ADHD—the presence of grandiosity, elated mood, and hypersexuality and, to a lesser extent, flights of ideas and decreased need for sleep. If one or more of these unique symptoms exists, you and your doctor should consider a diagnosis of bipolar disorder.

Depression

Children with bipolar disorder can have periods of mild or deep depression, so it is not uncommon that they are diagnosed and treated for depression. There are no easily reliable rules of thumb for differentiating unipolar depression from depression in bipolar disorder. However, if in the process of treating your child's depression, symptoms of mania or hypomania show up, consider a diagnosis of bipolar disorder.

Diagnosis can be especially tricky when the bipolar child has such mild manic symptoms that they are easily overlooked. This is a common problem with children diagnosed as bipolar II. It can be particularly hard to treat depression in bipolar disorder, as most medical interventions make bipolar disorder worse. During a depressive episode, children may be placed on antidepressant medication, but antidepressants generally aggravate bipolar symptoms, potentially setting off a manic episode. For example, I recently had a patient named Laura who came dressed in a pink fishnet top, showing several hallmarks of mania: rapid speech, hypervigilance, and irritability combined with flamboyance. She was accompanied by her mother, who was literally crying because this frightening change in behavior occurred after two doses of antidepressants. Even her 8-year-old brother said, "Mom, she was better off when she was depressed. Get her off the evil medication."

Behavior Disorders

Children with bipolar disorder share a number of behaviors with children who have behavior disorders such as ODD and CD. As bipolar kids can be defiant, irritable, and stubborn; get into arguments; become aggressive; fight; or run away, they are frequently diagnosed as having ODD or CD.

If a bipolar child is diagnosed with a behavior disorder and a therapist uses a behavior modification program with punishment as a consequence of undesired behavior, it can have a negative rather than positive effect. You know how little it takes to have your child slam the door and swear at you if you try to discipline her. In most cases, ODD is a "reactive" diagnosis—in other words, it occurs in response to a major upheaval or distressing symptoms of another disorder. It is hard to treat and resolves only months after treating the mood disorder. ODD is a comorbid condition only if it persists after the mood disorder is treated.

Behavior Disorders and Bipolar Disorder

Behavior only	Shared symptoms	Bipolar only
Persists after treatment of mood disorder; more family difficulties with major problems in style of parenting or family function; can be spiteful	Irritability Tantrums Defiance Disobedience	Behavior resolves, but slowly and after some months of treating the mood disorder; reactive, off-the-cuff acting out

Anxiety Disorders

A significant number (12–60%) of bipolar children are also diagnosed as having anxiety disorders, such as extreme separation anxiety, social phobias, generalized anxiety, panic disorder, or obsessive-compulsive disorder (OCD). These children develop maladaptive ways to deal with real or imagined fears, such as avoiding common social situations; developing physical symptoms such as headaches, stomachaches, or shortness of breath in response to worries; or developing uncontrollable repetitive thoughts or actions. Children who are exposed to traumatic experiences such as sexual abuse, neglect, or violence may develop symptoms of posttraumatic stress disorder (PTSD), including nightmares and flash-backs.

Anxiety symptoms are sometimes mistaken for bipolar disorder; for instance, children exhibit irritability, rages, and suicidal thoughts or state-ments in response to anxious thoughts. The opposite can be true as well. Manic symptoms can easily be mistaken for anxiety-related agitation or insomnia and, in fact, can be exacerbated by some anxiety medications. Diagnosing and appropriately treating these two sets of disorders—whether they are comorbid or not—requires careful evaluation and man-agement by a professional experienced in treating bipolar disorder and other psychiatric illnesses. An important point to note here is that where overfocused, intense, manic children ask incessantly to make phone calls or constantly ask to go shopping, parents sometimes wrongly believe it is OCD. This is intensity and pushy behavior seen in manic children and not OCD.

Other Diagnostic Complications

A number of other conditions produce symptoms that can resemble bipo-lar disorder and complicate diagnosis. For instance, substance abuse may induce hyper or risky behavior that resembles mania. In older adolescents, bipolar-induced delusions, hallucinations, and thought disorders can be mistaken for schizophrenia in up to 50% of cases. And the irritability, moodiness, and aggression sometimes seen in PDD or Asperger syndrome can also be mistaken for mania. Finally, some medical conditions such as premenstrual syndrome (PMS), thyroid disease, cancer, or reaction to cer-tain medications can trigger symptoms that resemble bipolar disorder. A thorough screening should take place to rule out any of these possibilities.

Getting the Right Diagnosis

It should be apparent at this point that an accurate diagnosis is one of the most important aspects of helping your child obtain appropriate and effec-tive treatment for bipolar disorder. But getting the right diagnosis can be tricky, especially when you factor in the wide variations in the way bipolar disorder manifests in different children at different developmental stages, the subtle variations in symptom clusters and subtypes, and the presence of "look-alike" conditions and/or comorbidities. Obviously, the potential for misdiagnosis, and consequently incorrect treatment, is huge. I want to encourage you to have a thorough evaluation if for any reason you are concerned about your child's diagnosis or feel that you need a second opinion to confirm what's going on.

It would be great if there was one end-all-be-all screening for bipolar disorder, but, sadly, this is not the case. We would all love to be able to look at a brain scan, give a blood test, or sequence a patient's genes and definitively rule out or confirm bipolar disorder. Perhaps, given the strides being made by medical researchers, someday that will be possible. In the meantime, however, bipolar disorder is diagnosed based on the presence of certain symptoms observed over a period of time, using various structured diagnostic tools and rating scales. For some children, it might even require hospitalization for a period of time. These diagnostic tools are evolving along with our understanding and the cumulative experience of doctors and families.

The other thing to remember is that your child's diagnosis may change over time as a result of changes in behavior and symptoms or because of new data coming to light. In other words, symptoms can change and evolve while your doctor gets to know your child and as your child develops. Thus, keep in mind that any diagnosis in the early stages of treatment should be viewed as a "working diagnosis." And finally, keep in mind that the diagnosis can also depend on the skill and experience of

---

Beware of Bogus Testing

Be cautious if someone wants to use actometers, telemetrics, and other gadgets to diagnose bipolar disorder or comorbid conditions, or encourages you to seek such tests. While these instruments may be potentially helpful, their use and interpretation can be skewed by self-interest, particularly if the practitioners have a business interest in the technology. For instance, some doctors may base a bipolar diagnosis on magnetic resonance imaging (MRI) findings alone rather than on a more comprehensive evaluation. Despite these limitations, some doctors go ahead and prescribe medication based on these test results. We have enormous respect for scientific development, but relying on such unproven tests at this stage and time may be a disservice to you and your child and may result in an unnecessary expense.

the doctor, so picking the right physician is a critical step, one that I discuss in more depth in Chapter 3.

What Are the Best Diagnostic Tools?

Several diagnostic tools are currently used to identify bipolar disorder. These instruments in most cases are designed to differentiate between bipolar disorder and look-alikes and/or comorbid conditions and are used in conjunction with a thorough clinical evaluation, which I will describe in detail below. The diagnostic tools generally involve semistructured interviews or "rating scales" administered by trained researchers, practitioners, and/or parents based on the type of instrument. The most commonly used of the research diagnostic tools are:

- The **Schedule for Affective Disorders and Schizophrenia (KSADS)** and the **Washington University KSADS (Wash-U-KSADS):** These assessments are usually administered in research settings and are free if they are undertaken as part of research. Be aware that they take 2 hours to complete and often are not necessary to make a clinical diagnosis. Tools really are as good as the clinicians who use them. These detailed interviews serve the researchers by allowing them to collect detailed information before they categorize children based on diagnosis, severity, and type of bipolar disorder, if they fall into that spectrum. These instruments do not replace good clinical training, and tools are not a substitute for bad training!
- The **Child Mania Rating Scale—Parent Version (CMRS-P):** This is a 21-item scale that I developed with my colleagues for completion by parents. A child who scores more than 20 on this scale is more than 90% likely to be diagnosed with bipolar disorder. The instrument is best used to alert parents to the possibility of bipolar disorder and should be confirmed by a good clinical evaluation. A sample of the parent version of this scale (CMRS-P) is included in Appendix B.

As I said earlier, as parents, you play a central role in diagnosing bipolar disorder. Many of these rating scales depend in whole or in part on parent reports. There's a good reason for this: parents often are the first to recognize and report signs of bipolar disorder. In a study comparing the screening potential of various rating scales, parents outperformed teacher reports and direct youth interviews for accurately recognizing bipolar disorder.

This just underscores what I said earlier about you as a parent sticking to your guns, even if everyone around you—your spouse, in-laws, a school administrator, even your doctor—doesn't believe you. You're not crazy, and it's not "all in your head"! Don't let them "blow you off" or accuse you of being "overprotective," as happens to so many parents in this situation. If you know there is a problem, try to find a qualified doctor who understands bipolar disorder and can provide a thorough evaluation and get you some answers. See Chapter 3 for more on finding qualified medical help.

What Does an Evaluation Involve?

While rating scales are promising, there is generally more to the evaluation process than a simple test can provide. One or more doctors, specialists, or paraprofessionals might become involved in completing a comprehensive evaluation. School psychologists, social workers, speech-language pathologists, or teachers might also weigh in, especially when you are getting appropriate educational placement and support for your child (see Chapter 9 for details).

Here are the general components of the evaluation:

Chief Complaints

All evaluations begin with meeting the parents to document a clear account of current problems, including examples of the sore points of daily life and how mood symptoms and functioning are affecting quality of life for your child and your family.

Social History

Factual background details are collected about the family structure, home environment, and the child's physical development, emotional history, school history, social life, hobbies, interests, challenges, and so on.

Psychological Evaluation

A comprehensive psychological evaluation should be performed by a qualified professional, a neuropsychologist if possible. The psychological evaluation includes several tests that measure intelligence, academic achievement levels, perceptual and language processing, and ability to complete tasks within a certain time frame. Occasionally, school districts dispute an outside psychological evaluation; even if they don't, many will still perform their own psychological evaluation in connection with educational placement.

Psychiatric or Neurological Evaluations

This evaluation should be done by an MD familiar with bipolar disorder, preferably a child psychiatrist or a general psychiatrist who is familiar with children. It should cover medical recommendations consisting of medications, therapy, counseling, and suggestions for home and school management. Be aware that no insurance adequately covers this, and it is often impossible to get one in a hurry because of doctors' busy schedules. Be prepared to pay extra to get this evaluation accomplished.

Education Evaluation

It is usually best for the school system to perform this battery of tests, which include spelling, decoding, writing, reading, comprehension, arithmetic, and mathematical word problems, if possible, though sometimes you may have to have it done by an outside evaluation team to get the school moving and to "prove" that your child has significant needs for which the school should provide services. Note that while schools are bound by federal law to provide accommodations for any child whose education would be hampered without them, they don't necessarily have to use outside evaluations at their expense, but can rely on their own. However, if parents pay to have a child evaluated for educational purposes, and the school doesn't have to pay for the outside evaluation, the school has to take the outside evaluators' findings into account.

Functional/Behavioral Assessment

Behavior management is usually a major issue for bipolar children, so this assessment will be very important for identifying your child's needs and the contextual factors that contribute to them, such as explosive tantrums or severe depressive spells. The last, but not least, component of this process is the development of a proposed pattern under which these behaviors usually occur, which can help pinpoint rapid cycling or severe mood fluctuations and identify any environmental triggers that could be involved. It is in this context that a narrative describing your observations of daily functioning, relationships with siblings and friends, and typical behavior at home and at school can be useful.

Evaluations for Comorbid Conditions

As discussed earlier in this chapter, it's common for a bipolar child to have coexisting conditions such as ADHD or another learning problem, for instance, difficulty with spelling, reading, writing, or arithmetic. He or she may also have problems processing language or following words and numbers on a page. A speech and language evaluation gives this type of information and determines whether additional services at school are needed, what kind, and how often they should be given. Anxiety disorders are very common comorbid conditions with bipolar disorder. A psychiatrist will become your best ally in helping sort out the complicated multilayered psychiatric disorders. In my opinion, a team evaluation at the diagnostic level is overkill. If the primary clinician is competent, too many cooks might spoil the broth. On the other hand, when a school is trying to determine any individualized education plan (IEP) or Section 504 needs of the child, occupational therapists, social workers, physiotherapists, and psychologists are needed at the school to help plan for and alleviate associated challenges.

Paying for the Evaluation

Knowing what your insurance plan allows and what type of services need preauthorization is critical. Every plan differs in the types of services that need preauthorization, from new psychiatric evaluations to lab work, so you need to be familiar with your plan. Many families fail to get preauthorization from their insurer for visits before they see a mental healthcare provider. In that case, the insurer can deny payment, resulting in huge out-of-pocket costs for services that might have been covered if preauthorization had been obtained. Remember to weigh carefully how your plan is working for your family at each benefits election period offered by your employer. Careful recordings of expenses, coverage, and hassles will help you determine if another choice may be more beneficial for your family.

Advocacy groups, such as the Child and Adolescent Bipolar Foundation, are working to pass an insurance parity bill that would require insurance companies to provide mental health coverage that is equivalent to the coverage offered for physical health care. This could affect how evaluations as well as treatment are paid for. To monitor the progress of this legislation and find out what it may mean for insurance coverage for childhood bipolar disorder, visit *bpkids.org*.

How Can You Help with Evaluation?

As a parent, you will play a central role as a source of information and facilitator of the evaluation process because you're the one who sees your child day in and day out, knows about the progression of the disease, and has information on previous diagnoses (or misdiagnoses) and treatment attempts.

You should be prepared to provide certain types of information on your child's history and symptoms as part of the evaluation process. Try to include:

1. Examples of difficult times, painting an authentic picture of what is going on. Include previous diagnoses (or misdiagnoses) and treatment attempts.
2. The nature of your child's mood fluctuations, based on the acronym FIND (Frequency, Intensity, Number, and Duration) of ups, downs, and mixed moods.
3. What you did to help, including a history of medications used; which ones helped and did not help; those that worsened symptoms and how. Include doses, duration used, and reasons for discontinuation (e.g., side effects).

To capture this information, you might keep a journal or use a worksheet. See the sample in Appendix D to see how you can compile the information in a useful form.

Finding the Right Professional Assistance

No matter where you are in the process of diagnosis and treatment, it's very important to choose the right doctor to work with over the long haul. This might be the same doctor who is involved in making your

You can be confident that the diagnostic process was adequate if, during the evaluation, you had a chance to:

1. Talk about all the worst experiences and the ebb and flow of symptoms over the years, leading up to the current time—that is, describe the "signature of the illness" as it presents in your child.
2. Specifically cover the mood symptoms—as you know them, at the minimum.
3. Let the doctor note the past medications used and responses to these medications.
4. Ask about school achievement and functioning.
5. Cover the family problems and stresses.
6. Discuss any associated psychiatric and medical disorders.
7. Go over the family history of any mental or physical disorders.
8. Feel understood as to the entire scenario, including symptom evolution and functioning.

Please note: Determining the accuracy of diagnosis is beyond the scope of any book and can be done only in person.

child's diagnosis, or it might be another doctor who steps in once the diagnosis is made because she is more readily available or better suited to your family's specific needs.

The next chapter explains how to choose a doctor and forge a good working relationship with him or her. It also explains the role that other practitioners can play in helping you and your family address bipolar disorder.

THREE

Finding the Right Doctor and Treatment Team

As your child and family's primary medical resource, your doctor is going to be the most critical member of the care team. The right doctor should make sure your child has the right diagnosis and spearhead the treatment plan as your child's situation changes and evolves. A supportive, knowledgeable physician can help you avoid medication mistakes and call in other specialists and relevant professionals needed to evaluate and treat your child and support the rest of the family.

Remember that doctors and other practitioners need parents' support and involvement in order to be effective. As I've mentioned elsewhere in this book, parents are the best source of information on what is happening with the bipolar child and should speak up about their needs. Gaining a good understanding of your child's disease and participating in her treatment and recovery is essential.

What Kind of Doctor Should You Look For?

Ideally, you will want to work with a child psychiatrist who is knowledgeable about bipolar disorder. It is possible that no child psychiatrists practice in your area. In that case, be prepared to work with an adult psychiatrist or a pediatrician who has experience with bipolar disorder. Although they are not specialists in children, general psychiatrists bring the advantage of knowing a lot about psychiatric medications; the downside can be that many still do not believe bipolar disorder exists in children. On the other hand, pediatricians better understand the physiology and development of children and can be more open to a bipolar diagnosis; pediatricians in remote areas can often work with experts in major medical centers in the nearest city to enhance your child's care. These generalities should be taken with a grain of salt. A lot depends on the training, personality, and willingness of the individual doctor, whose suitability should be evaluated on a case-by-case basis.

The sweetest doctor in the world could endanger your child's progress if he or she lacks knowledge of bipolar disorder. In this case, it makes sense to ask, "May I check with an expert and see if he or she will consult with us?" By the same token, a famous bipolar research expert may be brimming with knowledge but unavailable to you, so you might ask the expert to recommend someone who can respond to day-to-day crisis situations. Just as with your child, it is important to know what you might have to settle for and what you feel is an absolute requirement.

Where to Look for a Qualified Physician

Word of mouth from parents is sometimes the best avenue to locate a good doctor, but because of the sensitivities around mental illness in children, other parents may not put themselves forward as a resource. You also

---

Best Choices for Your Child's Primary Doctor (In Descending Order of Preference)

Child psychiatrist and expert in bipolar disorder
Child psychiatrist
Adult psychiatrist and expert in bipolar disorder
Adult psychiatrist
Advanced practice nurse and expert in bipolar disorder (rare, so lower on preference list)
Behavioral pediatrician
Pediatric neurologist
General pediatrician
Psychologists and social workers (need prescribing clinicians to be the partners in caring for the bipolar kids)

Links for Finding a Doctor

- Child and Adolescent Bipolar Foundation
  www.bpkids.org
- American Academy of Child and Adolescent Psychiatry
  www.aacap.org
- American Psychiatric Association
  www.psych.org
- National Alliance on Mental Illness
  www.nami.org
- Depression and Bipolar Support Alliance
  www.dbsalliance.org
- American Psychiatric Nurses Association
  www.apna.org
- American Psychological Association
  www.apa.org, 800-964-2000
- National Association of Social Workers
  www.socialworkers.org
- American Medical Association
  dbapps.ama-assn.org/aps/amahg.htm

---

may be reluctant to share information with other parents about your child's situation in this early stage for fear of labeling or stigmatization.

Fortunately, the Internet offers an easy, confidential alternative for locating a doctor, along with timely information and a virtual network of parents dealing with similar problems. One of the best resources on the Internet is the Child and Adolescent Bipolar Foundation (CABF), which maintains a listing of doctors by state at *www.bpkids.org*. Some excellent doctors who are not members of CABF will not be listed on the site, but you might be able to find them by visiting CABF chat rooms or posting a question on the message board. Other helpful websites include those of the National Alliance on Mental Illness (NAMI) at *www.nami.org* and Depression and Bipolar Support Alliance (DBSA) at *www.dbsalliance.org*. For a list of virtually all child psychiatrists in the United States, visit *www.aacap.org*.

If you don't have access to e-mail, you can use a computer at your local public library or get the help of a reference librarian to find addresses and phone numbers for these organizations.

Insurance Coverage and Your Physician

For most families today, insurance coverage is an important consideration and one that carries significant weight in the choice of doctors and other healthcare providers. As most people's insurance is provided through their employer, your choice of doctor will be affected by the type of plan and services your company offers or you choose (HMO, PPO, or FFS).

- In a health maintenance organization (HMO), your pediatrician is the gatekeeper for all specialty services and needs to be aware of services provided by specialists, so your providers are all aware of each other's involvement. Getting the referral form from the pediatrician to see a child psychiatrist or mental health specialist can be an obstacle. Families sometimes need to get several referrals over the course of their child's illness or may see a different doctor each time because the plan covers services from "any" in a particular managed care group. This can be frustrating and bears more importance when dealing with a child's emotion and behavior than with a sore throat. If you are not satisfied with the doctors in your plan, you are stuck. If you seek care outside of your HMO, you will likely have to pay full fees out of pocket.

- With a preferred provider organization (PPO), you can choose primary care and specialty care providers and see anyone on the list of providers without first obtaining a referral, but, even if you can locate a qualified doctor in your area, he or she may not be in your insurance network. The PPO may pay 100 or 90% of preferred providers' service charges but only 80 or 70% of an "out-of-network" provider's charges. One family I know found a great child psychiatrist in their area, but he stopped taking their insurance. Because it is so important to them, they now drive 70 miles to a pediatric neurologist who understands bipolar disorder and medications. In some PPOs, families handle claims; in others, doctors' offices may also take care of paperwork. Out-of-pocket expenses are typically higher in PPOs; they may involve more paperwork, but they do offer choice.

- In a fee-for-service (FFS) arrangement, the doctor bills the family for a service, and the family pays the entire bill, then submits it to the insurance company for reimbursement. You must know your out-of-pocket expenses in advance, so that, if your insurance only reimburses 50% of a $90 visit, you know in advance that out-of-pocket expenses will be $45. This can be hard for families who have difficulties paying cash up front and when reimbursements can take up to several weeks. When a child is being seen frequently, this can add up to a lot of up-front costs. Also, insurance companies may reimburse for visits but have a cap on how much they can reimburse. As always, you need to know your plan allows for mental health services before you seek them and be ready to ask about specialists rather than generalists. Although there are typically fewer restrictions with this type of plan, there is certainly more paperwork and less assistance with finding providers than with other plans.

Insurance can be such a critical issue that some families change insurance providers, switch jobs, or move to different cities to be able to work with a particular doctor over the long-term. Others may opt to pay out of pocket to obtain expert care. But moving, changing jobs, leaving a familiar neighborhood, or paying out of pocket can create significant hardships for many families. Only you can decide how much you and your family are able to sacrifice in other parts of your lives to obtain the help your bipolar child needs. (Later in this chapter, I talk about insurance coverage for therapists and the other practitioners your child may end up seeing.)

Checking Credentials and Training

As soon as you identify one or more doctors available to work with you, it's a good idea to do an Internet search to find out more about them, such as where they went to medical school, when they graduated, and where they completed residency. It is a plus if these doctors are licensed therapists or have obtained board certification in general and child psychiatry. If you don't find pertinent information on the Internet, it is perfectly all right to call each practice and ask the staff a few questions about the doctor's experience and training in diagnosing and treating bipolar disorder, the type of treatment she provides, and similar information. Staff might not be able to answer all these questions, and it can be awkward to ask some of these questions over the phone in advance. You might be better off asking your doctor about his credentials at the first office visit, but approach it sensitively and in a respectful tone so as not put him on the defensive. See the box on the facing page for a few examples of phrases that will enhance your interaction with prospective doctors.

Physician Interview Dos and Don'ts

Don't say . . .	Do say . . .
"Do you believe in childhood bipolar disorder or not?"	"What do you think causes these problems in children?"
"Why don't you believe my assessment of the situation?"	"I often think the problem is ×; what do you think?"
"Do you have enough experience with bipolar kids?"	"How long have you been seeing these types of kids?"
"What is your success rate?"	"You see a lot of these kids . . . do they get any better?"

One cautionary note about credentials: For a variety of reasons, many excellent doctors don't pursue board certification. At the same time, some board-certified physicians are not good at treating bipolar disorder, so take these credentials with a grain of salt. The most important thing is the doctor's knowledge and experience with bipolar disorder and his or her ability to relate to you and your child. Trust your instincts!

How to Choose the Right Doctor

Once you have determined the type of doctor you need and researched one or more qualified, affordable possibilities in your area, the next step is finding the doctor who is both qualified to treat bipolar disorder in children and able to connect well with you and your family. The only way to know for sure is to meet the doctor and speak with him, and it may take meeting with more than one doctor before you discover someone with the right mix of capabilities and personal qualities that signal a good fit.

Any parent of a child with this condition can tell stories of seeking out a second, third, or fourth doctor because the previous one(s) did not understand or could not help. When a search for help bogs down or fails, families are understandably discouraged, but the process can be easier if you start your search with two basic criteria in mind: the doctor–diagnosis fit and the doctor–family fit.

Doctor–Diagnosis Fit

Although bipolar disorder has been identified as a legitimate and autonomous illness for centuries and children with the disorder long have been described in case reports, research about the disorder in children has evolved in only the last decade. As a result, some physicians accept and understand pediatric bipolar disorder, but some remain skeptical or simply do not believe the disorder exists in childhood because it manifests so differently from adult bipolar disorder. You can save a lot of time and money and avoid stress if you ask up front whether a doctor believes that bipolar disorder can and does exist in children. "Despite a strong family history of bipolar disorder and the fact that my son met the criteria," said one mother, "he was put on antidepressants and got extremely manic and out of control. I think the doctor didn't believe kids could have bipolar disorder." According to another parent, "You want to trust the professionals, but they don't really know sometimes what to do. The behavioral pediatrician just throws meds around and has trouble keeping up with everything we have tried." Ideally, your child's doctor should be aware of the fledgling stage of research in the field and open to the idea of pediatric bipolar diagnosis. Sadly, it is quite common to hear parents say they wish they could have found a doctor willing and able to diagnose their child from the beginning.

Doctor–Family Fit

Your relationship with your child's doctor is extremely important. Many families come to our clinic after having visited several doctors without getting effective help—even getting a diagnosis can be a struggle. In fact, we believe that, as a result of these bad experiences, some families have a hard time at first trusting that help is at hand. Even the children feel the stress. One child told his parent, "No one is trying to help me but you and Daddy. My brain just won't work right."

Thus, you are looking for a doctor who will treat you and your opinion with respect. He should clearly convey his belief that your role is essential, even central, to the overall success of your child's treatment plan. This includes listening to your input and taking seriously your feedback and observations about your child and his or her needs.

A doctor who is willing to partner with you will include you in decision making and consider your needs as parents in delivering the treatment directly or by arranging additional help. She should also support your central role by helping you evolve as a coach in managing your child's care while validating your own needs as you adjust to this new role.

As mentioned earlier, if your doctor clearly doesn't believe you, accuses you of misrepresenting your child's symptoms, or dismisses useful information you provide, he may not be the right doctor for your family, regardless of his expertise and experience.

What does it take to develop a trusting relationship with your child's doctor? Like any relationship, it requires time and effort on both sides. For your part, it helps if you clearly communicate your expectations and give your doctor regular feedback about how well she is doing helping your family. To treat the disease effectively, you need to be able to tell your doctor, "that's working well," or "we need more help with this problem." As a general rule, doctors, like anyone else, want to do a good job and want to be appreciated for it. A good relationship is also a two-way street. Just as you should listen carefully to your doctor and try to understand and follow what she is telling you, your doctor should also be willing to listen

---

Tips for Maximizing Your Relationships with Your Doctor

- Participate and be proactive in reaching for help!
- Speak up about all your problems.
- Provide information, such as the nature (FIND—frequency, intensity, number, and duration of symptoms) *of the illness, medications and other treatments that have been tried, and reasons for making changes.*
- Know your rights. For more information on rights of individuals with psychiatric disorders, see NAMI and your state's mental health code.
- Get the facts and learn as much as you can.
- Remember that parents are experts too; believe in yourself.
- Recognize efforts by professionals and remember that all humans thrive on positive interaction.
- Communicate clearly and assertively. If you feel you have not been understood, be persistent and patient. Try to rephrase your point calmly, or write it down and bring it to the next session. No matter what happens, raising your voice or using a curt or demanding tone is inadvisable and could damage your long-term relationship with your doctor.

to and rely on you to provide clear and specific reports about the nature and quantity of your child's symptoms and how they manifest in all aspects of your child's life.

Interviewing Prospective Doctors

Your first meeting with a prospective doctor for your child should be approached like an interview, but move toward building a bridge if things go well. You should take control of the meeting in your head by coming prepared with questions such as the ones in the box below and stating what you believe you and your child need from the doctor or clinician. Don't be worried at this stage about whether your requests are realistic or whether the doctor can meet them. The important thing is to check for a few basic clues as to whether the doctor has the right mix of expertise and

---

Questions to Ask When You Interview a Doctor

- Can you help me understand bipolar disorder in children better? How do you make your diagnosis?
- What do you think it will take for my child to get better?
- What types of treatment do you or your staff offer children with bipolar disorder?
- What is the prognosis for these types of kids? Do kids get better in your experience? How long does it take to see changes? And what changes can I expect?
- How long does treatment usually take? Does it mean lifelong medication? How much do I get to be part of the treatment?
- Will my other kids get to see you to discuss their worries and concerns? Can you recommend other therapists to help them?
- How often can we see you? Or need to see you?
- We live far away—is it possible to work with our hometown doctor, who is open to working with you?
- Can we reach you between sessions, and how (phone, e-mail)? Are you available to participate in an IEP teleconference? Do you charge for the phone calls? (This last question can be answered by assistants.)
- What kind of crises can I expect that might require me to call you?
- Are you affiliated with an inpatient psychiatric facility should the need arise?

You want to work with a doctor who . . .

1. **Has good interpersonal skills:** Greets you and your children in a warm, welcoming manner and is interested in hearing what you have to say. The doctor should express empathy and demonstrate a caring attitude. Avoid a grumpy or argumentative doctor who won't let you offer new information, voice your opinions, or confirm what you have learned. Although you may not know the latest in evidence-based practices, you should feel comfortable asking questions and sharing what you have learned!

2. **Respects the parent's role:** Listens, respects, and tunes in to what you have to say and treats you as a valued member in your child's care team. When talking with the doctor, you should feel like a collaborator, rather than patronized as just another "case."

3. **Communicates in clear, simple terms:** Uses everyday language to explain bipolar disorder, mood regulation, medications, and common interpersonal conflicts. He or she should use terms that even your child can understand. Some doctors use scientific "mumbo jumbo" as a defense. A smart doctor uses simple language!

4. **Understands treatment options:** Understands bipolar-specific psychotherapy techniques and their use in conjunction with medications. The complexity of a bipolar diagnosis calls for complex types of treatment, often more complex than managing medications!

5. **Cares for the whole family:** Bipolar disorder has an impact on the entire family, and every member needs help coping with the effects of this illness on her life. The doctor should appreciate your struggles as a parent and show interest in helping *you.* He should also involve siblings in treatment, gently helping them understand the disorder while equipping them to cope (for more on this subject, see Chapter 8).

6. **Respects other professionals:** Your doctor should be able and willing to work with other specialists and healthcare professionals to provide the best care for your child. A pediatrician or a doctor in a remote setting should consult with an expert or an able child psychiatrist, if needed. A doctor who speaks disparagingly of peers may reflect her own limitations and fears and be less able to offer your child what he needs. "We had great doctors who tried so hard to help," a parent relates. "Our pediatrician did all he could, then sent us on to a child neurologist. The neurologist ran tests, and diagnosed him with ADHD/ODD at around age 5. From there she sent us to a child psychiatrist. We also went to alternative doctors. We had him tested for all kinds of things, including mineral and vitamin deficiencies. We took him for occupational therapy for a while too. Nothing

(cont.)

(cont.)

seemed to really work. After 3 years with the psychiatrist, she finally diagnosed him with bipolar/ADHD."

7. **Instills a sense of hope:** Is positive, hopeful, and committed to helping you and your child succeed. The colors of your child's moods are beautiful like a rainbow, but the extremes need modulating.

8. **Is available:** The doctor should be willing to provide options, strategies, tips, and tricks beyond the prescription pad to help you and your child succeed.

personal qualities to work well with you and your family, summarized in the sidebar on pages 57–58.

Getting Off on the Right Foot with Your Doctor

Now that you have chosen a doctor, it's important to set the stage for a positive working relationship from the beginning. If you haven't already obtained a diagnosis, your doctor should begin with a comprehensive evaluation of your child and, based on that assessment, provide a diagnosis, along with the reasoning behind the diagnosis. The doctor should also offer an estimate of your child's prognosis, or a prediction of how your child might fare over the course of development.

Records and Notes to Keep on Hand and Take to Your Doctor's Visit

In preparation for seeing a doctor, make checklists and notes about your child. Jot down things to discuss with the doctor; list things you need to cope with and things the doctor might be able to do to help you and your family function better (such as helping siblings with therapy or providing access to a support group through the clinic). This will come in handy, especially in a crisis. Organize elements such as mood charts, medication histories, patterns of illness episodes, and positive effects you want to show your doctor. We also recommend that parents keep a special journal—collect pieces of information and string your own inspiring statements together like pearls.

Make a list of all the books you have read on subjects related to your child's mood and behavior. Revisit key points that most impressed you by rereading each book and highlighting aspects that appeal to you. It may also help to write notes on these key points in your journal. They may serve as special jewels you consult or read when you feel disillusioned or stuck. You can make flash cards to help you cover important matters while at the doctor's office or to use when you are in distress or are facing complicated situations with your child. Your journal will be useful in good times and hard times, and take-away tools such as flash cards help make your journal portable. You may often feel you have lost direction or progress. In such times, try to make a list of simple, bite-sized goals. Recording progress and your own goals and needs will create a tool to help support more meaningful talk with your doctor and will help you stay focused on the bigger vision when an episode of illness throws you off course. Think of what you need in your treasure chest and begin planning and stocking it today.

Being Prepared for Doctor's Visits

It's hard to remember everything you want to talk to the doctor about, but any or all of these tools can help you make the most of your time at doctor's visits.

- A list of questions that have come up since your last doctor's visit. Some parents make flash cards to remind them of what they absolutely must cover on a particular visit.
- A list of problems you need to cope with. You can chip away at this list by bringing up your top priorities at the first visit and then working your way through the list at subsequent visits.
- A folder for mood charts (if you're using them; see Chapter 6).
- A folder for medication histories with any notes on positive effects and side effects your child has experienced with different drugs.
- A list of other strategies (such as RAINBOW strategies; see Chapter 6) that you've found particularly helpful to your child.
- A list of very specific, attainable goals (break down larger goals, like "Establish a good sleep routine," into smaller ones, like "Get Jenny to bed 15 minutes earlier every night this week" and "Find a bedtime story that's soothing and relaxing") that the doctor can advise you on reaching.

**Tools You Can Use to Keep Yourself on Track—
and on an Even Keel**

You'll find many of the tools in Chapter 8 just as helpful to you at home as in communicating with your child's doctors. In addition, the following can give you opportunities to reflect, learn from your experiences, and make a personal habit of the positive self-talk that you'll be encouraging your child to adopt (see Chapter 6).

- A journal that you use to record your hopes, dreams, and fears for your child, with highlights on thoughts you want to remember when you reread entries later.
- Books you've found helpful, with highlighted passages so that you don't later forget messages that helped you when you first read them. The books I like the best are listed in the Resources.
- Note cards with important principles and self-coaching thoughts that you can carry around with you and turn to when a crisis arises and you feel overwhelmed.

Working with Your Doctor during Treatment

Your child's doctor should be able to warn you off the latest faddish explanations for bipolar disorder and spare you the expense and time wasted chasing bogus testing or treatment. Beware any explanation or treatment option based on questionable or controversial research. Typically, research that is published in reputable, academic journals or reviewed by leaders in the field will offer more science-based treatments than that discussed only by word of mouth or in nonscientific publications.

It is critical that you have some understanding of your doctor's philosophy, approach to treatment, and decision-making process. The treatment plan should take into account the biological, psychological, and family factors of child, parent, and school system. The strengths and weaknesses of each factor should be considered in treatment decisions. This part of the assessment is often called a "formulation" in psychiatric terms.

Doctors frequently are pressed for time, but at minimum you can expect the doctor to draw a flowchart or Venn diagram of all the issues or priorities in treatment. Part of the education process at this point is to inform the family of the main areas of focus for treatment and what to expect in outcome to track changes. Outcome is not straightforward and is fraught with trials and errors in treatment, encumbered with barriers, and framed within an eventual hope of recovery.

We frequently hear families say things such as "The doctor insisted that our child had ADHD and had to be medicated for it before he could do anything else," or "The doctors diagnosed his depression and insisted on prescribing antidepressants, which we knew would make our child's symptoms worse. It did and he ended up in the hospital." Having explanations for treatment decisions will keep you, your child, and your doctor engaged in the treatment process and ensure that everyone understands his or her roles and responsibilities.

Your doctor should also explain the goal, format, and delivery of each technique used in the treatment plan—who will deliver a service (for instance, a family therapist or child psychologist), who will receive it, and in what time frame. Once you have some insight into your doctor's decision-making process, you will also better understand why your child is completing a particular course of therapy, what to expect from a specific medication, and where the treatment will go next if this approach does not work.

Be wary of complicated plans that have no "teeth" in the process or options that are unrealistic for your situation. For example, if you live in a rural area that has no therapists skilled in helping bipolar children, prescribing child- and family-focused cognitive therapy may not be reasonable. Even if a wide range of practitioners is available to you, your child and family may not need to pull out every stop and waste your time and tire your child for no good reason! The plan should be designed to fit the child, the family, and the situation. For instance, if a family is already communicating well with their child and managing her behavior at home, we would focus treatment on improving the child's experience with school and friends. Or if a family is working with an inexperienced local practitioner, our team might focus instead on introducing the doctor to important treatment principles and sharing appropriate clinical information.

The treatment plan proposed by the doctor should . . .

- be evidence-based—that is, supported by scientific research and a wealth of clinical experience.
- take into account strengths and weaknesses of the child, family, and school system.

- list priorities and focus of treatment, plus how improvements will be tracked.
- specify who will deliver each part of treatment, who (child or other family members) will receive it, and over what time frame.
- specify what will be tried next if treatments don't work.
- be realistically accessible to your family.

NOTE: As you read this book, remember to think about how these general principles relate to your own situation and jot down notes as to how you could apply them to your child's and family's challenges. That way, you can incorporate the ideas into your daily experience, rather than simply try to absorb them through reading.

Managing Medications Together

It is hard to understand the complexities in prescribing medication and to feel confident that your doctor will arrive at the right combination, particularly if your child has had bad experiences with medication in the past. Your doctor should provide information about medications for your child, what to expect from medications, why certain medications are chosen, and the logic behind the medications or combinations of drugs being prescribed. If selective serotonin reuptake inhibitors (SSRIs) and stimulant medications have harmed your child in the past, or you know that other medications have not worked in the past, it is important that you share that information with your doctor so you can avoid unnecessary crises or loss of valuable treatment time.

In addition, pharmaceutical companies and medical centers provide information on various medications used to treat bipolar disorder. In Chapter 5, I go into detail about how medication will be used to manage your child's moods. In addition, for easy reference, I have included a list of the most commonly prescribed medications with an overview about how they work and likely side effects in Chapter 5 and a list of medications in Appendix F.

Reaching Your Doctor in a Crisis

Once the treatment plan is laid out, it is extremely important to establish how to intervene in a crisis. This includes educating parents about signs of crises versus the rough spots and glitches that inevitably occur and how to recognize which is which. Discuss with your doctor what constitutes a crisis and how you both should respond to anticipated problems. In your first or second session, be sure to ask your doctor, "If I have questions between visits, what is the best way to address them?" and "If there is a crisis, what is the best way to reach you?" While it is important not to contact your doctor about every small problem, you should have contact information and permission to call in times of true crisis.

There may be times when your doctor won't be able to respond immediately or fully to your needs because of the demands of other patients, the doctor's institution or practice, or even his or her own family. Nevertheless, you may need access to medical support 24 hours a day, 7 days a week! Some questions may be easily answered by the doctor's office staff, but others may need the doctor's personal attention. It is important to be conscious of these levels of care and your doctor's arrangements for them.

Monitoring and Follow-Up

Regular visits, careful monitoring, and follow-up are essential components of long-term quality care. Your doctor should see your child and you at least one or two times to make an initial diagnosis or confirm a diagnosis made elsewhere. Parents often wonder if doctors should "label" a child after seeing him only once. Of course, no one is completely foolproof and human errors are inevitable, but usually clinicians are trained to understand problems in a short period of time and one session is appropriate to come up with a working diagnosis.

While it is routine to see new patients every 2 to 3 weeks at the beginning of treatment, depending on the distance and difficulties of travel, a less intensive schedule could be warranted. It takes roughly 4 to 6 months to stabilize symptoms in a typical complicated case, and complexity is the rule, rather than the exception, given the high probability of secondary issues such as ADHD, depressive symptoms, sleep difficulties, medication side effects, and psychosis due to breakthrough symptoms of mania.

Your doctor should have an adequate repertoire of tools to record symptoms and checklists to monitor medication side effects. This repertoire should also include knowledge of laboratory tests, diagnostic tests, and measures for tracking outcomes. Your doctor should be familiar with when and why tests should be completed and should help you and your child know what to expect and when and how to measure your successes at a clinical level. The doctor should be able to supply you with a mood chart that serves as a visual analogue or checklists for you to complete, such as the Child Mania Rating Scale (CMRS), the Pediatric Side Effects Checklist (P-SEC), or a checklist of medications with outcome ratings from past history (to give a bird's-eye view of what has been tried). Samples of these tools are in included in Appendices B, D, and E. Feel free to copy them and even supply them to your doctor if needed. Keep in mind that tools are sexy but will not or cannot replace the clinical acumen and valuable experience of a good psychiatrist.

Administrative Resources to Request from Your Doctor

Record and Reports

Your child's doctor(s) should provide you with a written report for your own records. In today's mobile society, documentation of tests and evaluations is essential, as it can save you the expense of repeating earlier tests and enhance the quality of future care, as healthcare providers will be able to determine exactly what has and has not been done.

Letters of Support or Other Communications

Your child's doctor(s) should be prepared to supply various letters of support and other documentation of your child's problems upon request to help ensure that your child's needs are addressed in all settings. The doctor(s) should proactively contact schools and be available for teleconferencing or providing letters of support, write short notes to therapist(s) and teachers to advocate for services, and outline problems and solutions or provide anticipatory information to summer camps or others who are important in your child's care. It may not be realistic to expect a busy doctor to deliver this care in person, but the office staff might be able to help with some of these needs.

Working with Other Specialists and Practitioners

In addition to your doctor, a number of other practitioners are likely to be involved in your child's evaluation, diagnosis, and treatment program, such as nurse practitioners, physicians' assistants, psychologists, therapists, social workers, speech and language specialists, occupational therapists (for handwriting problems), and more.

In some cases, these professionals may provide primary care in the absence of an available qualified medical doctor. In our clinic, some families come from areas hundreds of miles away where there are no child psychiatrists or doctors experienced in treating bipolar disorder. In these cases, especially in the early phases of mood stabilization, we write down guidelines based on evidence-driven pharmacotherapy for bipolar disorder and offer to talk with the collaborating physician between sessions as needed.

Since medication management is likely to be part of your child's care, it is important to choose someone who is able to prescribe or is able to work closely with a prescribing professional. In some cases, advanced practice nurses (or nurse practitioners) and physicians' assistants can function as doctors. Other clinicians, such as psychologists, clinical social workers, or therapists, who cannot prescribe medications are also very useful for behavioral management and psychotherapy, which are discussed in more detail in Chapter 6. Consider yourself fortunate if your therapist and prescriber are the same person.

When Is Consultation or Referral Needed?

Your doctor should be willing to ask for help from other doctors and to refer you to other specialists as needed. Depending on your child's age (some of these issues will be more relevant to preteens and those entering puberty), consultation or referral to other specialists might include neurologists (to rule out epilepsy or neurological causes), dermatologists (for acne that may emerge with lithium), gynecologists (medication-related problems such as menstrual irregularities, hormonal elevations such as with prolactin that may occur with risperidone, or ovarian cysts that can be caused by valproate), and endocrinologists (for high thyroid-stimulating hormone sometimes seen with lithium) as needed.

Be mindful of your primary doctor's comfort level with receiving advice (at times, it amounts to a second opinion), and be aware that some experts may be disinclined to give direct, unsolicited advice. You as parent can best judge whether to request a direct dialogue between the two physicians or to act as a middleman. In an ideal world, there should be a free flow of information focused on your child's health and well-being without interference from egos and professional jealousies.

Glossary of Practitioner Types

- **Advanced practice nurse:** a registered nurse with a master's or doctorate in nursing with certification who evaluates and treats children and adults with emotional and behavioral disorders. Can prescribe medication.
- **Child and adolescent psychiatrist:** a medical doctor (MD), who has completed training as a physician in general psychiatry, plus training in child and adolescent psychiatry. Can prescribe medication and do therapy.
- **Child psychologist:** a psychologist with a doctorate (PhD or PsyD) who specializes in children and adolescents. See "clinical psychologist" below.
- **Clinical psychologist, psychologist:** a mental health provider with a doctorate (PhD or PsyD) in psychology who tests, evaluates, and treats children and adults with emotional and behavioral disorders. Cannot prescribe medication.
- **Clinical social worker:** a mental health provider with a master's (MSW) or doctorate (PhD) in social work who evaluates and treats children and adults with emotional and behavioral disorders. Cannot prescribe medication.
- **EdD:** a person with a doctorate in education. Sometimes does psychotherapy.
- **LCSW:** a licensed clinical social worker (a mental health professional with a master's degree in social work (MSW) as well as advanced clinical experience and licensure in his or her specialty area.
- **MD:** a person with a doctorate in medicine. Can prescribe medication. Includes pediatricians, psychiatrists, neurologists, and family practitioners.
- **MSW** a master's degree in social work.
- **Neuropsychologist:** a person who does comprehensive testing on cognitive abilities like IQ, attention, academic ability, etc.
- **Pediatrician:** a medical doctor (MD) who specializes in treating all types of childhood illnesses.
- **PhD:** indicates that a person has a doctoral degree, usually in psychology.
- **Physician's assistant (PA):** a person with special training, less than an MD, but able to treat and prescribe medication under an MD's supervision.
- **Psychiatric nurse:** a registered nurse (RN) who specializes in treating children and adults with emotional or behavioral disorders.

- **Psychiatrist:** a medical doctor (MD) who specializes in psychiatry; able to treat children and adults with emotional or behavioral disorders. Can prescribe medication.
- **Psychopharmacologist:** an MD experienced in the use of psychiatric medications. Unfortunately, many MDs are not fully skilled in this area.
- **Therapist:** any professional who provides psychotherapy.

Paying for a Therapist

Because bipolar disorder is a chronic and episodic illness, it is important to know yearly visit caps, out-of-pocket maximums, hospitalization and partial hospitalization coverage (days), substance abuse coverage, and yearly and lifetime maximums. To get the most out of whatever coverage you do have, you should be aware of the following:

- *Know the rules:* Beware of some typical errors in using your insurance plans! Many families fail to get preauthorization from their insurer before they see a mental healthcare provider. In that case, the insurer can deny payment, resulting in huge out-of-pocket costs for services that might have been covered if preauthorization had been obtained. Knowing what your plan allows and what type of services need preauthorization is critical. Every plan differs in the types of services that need preauthorization, from new psychiatric evaluations to lab work.
- *Know the limits:* Each new calendar year begets a rash of changes in deductible requirements, coverage ceilings, and requirements for reevaluating your child's illness and treatment. Families need to know how to spend their allocated yearly visits (typically 20 per calendar year) and how to make the most of those visits over the year. For instance, some clinicians may insist that you see them weekly, but you may be able to stretch time between visits if your child is fairly stable. Or, perhaps the family benefits most from counseling sessions with the child's therapist and needs fewer medication adjustments than last year. Of course, if you decide to reduce the frequency of your visits, make sure you know how to reach your provider between visits if needed.
- *Know your options:* Some insurance companies count a course of group therapy as equivalent to a certain number of family or individual therapy visits. In these cases, you may be able to stretch your visit allow-

ance by using group therapy for your child, but make sure it is good, empirically based, and child-appropriate therapy. The catch here may be the availability of appropriate groups that are suitable for these children and the groups that allow space for a bipolar kid. The best groups are those that address some of these things if not all of them: mood regulation, anger control, social skills and friendship building skills, problem solving, communication skills, and building self-esteem. Talk honestly with your mental health provider about these very real issues, so you can devise a strategy to use your visits wisely.

Saving for a rainy day is sort of what flexible spending accounts (FSAs) for medical expenses are to families. These accounts help families put aside pre-tax income in an account specifically for medical costs. Many families save hundreds of dollars using these accounts, due to the pre-tax benefit. Check to see if your employer covers these types of plans during your next benefits enrollment period. Be aware that generally, if you don't use all the money in an FSA in a given calendar year, you lose it. There are also caps on how much you can put in one.

When to Consider Finding Another Practitioner

I don't like the idea of doctor shopping—it causes a lot of disruption and instability for you and your child, which is the last thing you need; however, I recommend that you consider a change when the doctor's treatment approach is hurting more than helping, or when you feel stuck, uncomfortable, and resentful. You don't need more stress in your life beyond having to cope with a bipolar child! Most of the time, any difficulties can be resolved, especially in cases of simple misunderstandings or oversights. But if the problems listed below do not disappear after a brief discussion, there may be a personality conflict or a strong difference in philosophy, or the practitioner may not have the level of expertise needed to manage your child's care. It's time to find a new clinician. When you believe the diagnostic process was incomplete or inaccurate and the diagnosis does not align with your intuition, observations, or other informed opinions, a new doctor may be needed. This is especially true if you did not have a chance to discuss the findings and come to a mutual understanding.

What do you do if a practitioner keeps information from parents based on the "confidentiality" of the child?

Any child under age 17 is considered a minor, which means you not only have to give your permission for your child to receive treatment, but you also have a right to receive all information about the treatment your child gets. As trust is so important to a fruitful relationship between doctor and patient, most doctors and therapists (including me) talk to the family ahead of time to ensure that both parents and child understand some things will be kept private at the child's request *if* they don't involve the child's safety and *if* sharing the information with parents doesn't seem crucial to solving a problem involved with a treatment goal. *If your child admits to suicidal thoughts or wishes to harm someone else, any clinician who gains this information must share it with you.*

As a clinician, here's how I tend to handle these situations: If the child tells me that she is having trouble with a sibling or at school and asks me not to reveal it to her parents, I will size up the situation carefully. I wouldn't overreact nor would I minimize the child's feelings. I might encourage the child to talk it over with her parents or to work through her anger by role-playing with me. I would gently ask her parents to keep an eye out for potential sibling or school conflicts without sharing the specific details of the child's comments. Not to minimize the risk, but there is often a lot of drama with these kids. I use my clinical judgment to discern whether there is a serious risk or whether this is just an expression of a volatile, rageful child.

Please note that as your child approaches adolescence, it's likely that privacy will become a greater issue, and renewed discussion of the ground rules between the doctor/therapist and the whole family may be wise.

- When you believe that one or more elements of the treatment plan are ineffective, counterproductive, or damaging. Examples might include your observation that a medication isn't making a difference or, in the case of stimulants or antidepressants, is worsening the clinical state.
- When the practitioner won't change the treatment plan or adjust the dosing level to match the child's growth and development.
- When the practitioner doesn't seem concerned about worsening

symptoms or a possible relapse despite your alerting him or her to the fact.

- When you have not received satisfactory explanations for treatment and medication recommendations, there are gaps or inconsistencies in the information the doctor provides that you can't seem to reconcile, and you and your spouse have questions that the practitioner doesn't have the expertise or information to answer.
- When the practitioner is not communicating or collaborating with you or other professionals in the context of serious problems across settings where intervention is essential to dispel misunderstandings.
- When the doctor doesn't relate to problems at school or in other spheres of the child's life.
- When the practitioner can't treat comorbid conditions and doesn't make appropriate referrals.
- When therapy doesn't seem to be helping.

Reaching for the RAINBOW

If your child has already been diagnosed with bipolar disorder, I hope the chapters in Part I have given you the confidence that the diagnostic process was thorough and expert, the physician and other practitioners are the best ones you can find for your child and your family, and you know what treatment should aim for to produce the best outcome for your son or daughter. If you haven't completed this process yet, I hope you feel better equipped to pursue this important preliminary step. Once you've done so, you can get started on the treatment that combines the benefits of medication, therapy, and skilled parenting to help your child and your family reach for the best possible future for all.

PART II

Treatment That Can Help Your Child and Your Family

FINDING THE SOLUTIONS

Understanding bipolar disorder and finding professionals who can help your child is a big step in a long journey that will change and evolve as your child grows. Your circumstances may change as well, so how you treat the disorder may have to change, too. In addition, the state of scientific knowledge is rapidly evolving, new medications are being developed and tested, and doctors and families are learning more about what works every day—there's no telling what new and improved treatment approaches could emerge in the future.

For the time being, however, the basic tools for treating bipolar disorder in children consist of medication combined with psychotherapy and behavior management. I will address each of these subjects in detail in the next few chapters. My own approach combines medication management with child- and family-focused cognitive-behavioral therapy (CFF-CBT; RAINBOW therapy) that incorporates interpersonal therapy as well, a treatment plan we've named Multi-Modal Integrated Therapy for Youth with Bipolar Disorder (MITY-BD). Based on a model used with bipolar adults, this combination has been shown in research and clinical practice to give children and families the best chance of success for treating bipolar disorder. While RAINBOW therapy and MITY-BD are unique to our university clinic, the principles behind them can be readily integrated into any treatment program that combines medication management with a psychotherapeutic approach. So, even if you can't find a doctor who offers the exact same program in your community, you can share this philosophy and tools with your doctors and therapists and use these principles to help manage bipolar disorder at home. It is unrealistic for me to expect you to have access to a trained therapist if you live, for example, in a rural area with no doctor, let alone therapist, for miles around you.

Even with the best-case scenario, treatment will continue to be challenging. Anyone who has ever dealt with bipolar disorder as a patient, a family member, or a professional knows that day-to-day management can be pretty complicated. It takes patience, trial and error, and close monitoring to come up with the specific combination of levers and pulleys that work in your child's and family's case. And just when you think you've got it down—bam! Something changes, and you've got to go through the process once again.

Yes, it's hard, but it's not hopeless. There is a "rainbow" after the storm, as you will see, if you approach the problem in a way that involves the whole family and integrates the various strategies into a program that addresses this complex disorder in its many hues and shades.

FOUR

Setting the Stage to Make the Most of Treatment

PRINCIPLES TO GET YOU OFF TO A GOOD START

"He is having conversations, interested in what others have to say, listens, drawing complete pictures instead of disjointed scribbles. We can go to restaurants now . . . by no means is he an easy kid, but very manageable after we started treatment."

This is the kind of transformation every parent of a bipolar child hopes for but fears will never take place. I want to assure you that it is possible and that you and your child can have a better, more manageable life. To get there, you need to have some basic tools at your disposal, the right kind of professional support, and some realistic operating principles that can help you and your child get on and stay on the path to success. As much as you may wish, you can't just take a little of this and a little of that, stir them together, and expect it to work, work every time, or work forever. But there are some basic ingredients—a recipe for success, if you will—that produce the best outcomes for your child.

Why Child- and Family-Focused Cognitive-Behavioral Therapy (CFF-CBT)?

Before I get into the specific components of medication (Chapter 5) and therapy (Chapter 6), I want to help you establish a good foundation for your child's treatment. Brick by brick, we're going to build an unshakable structure to support your child's treatment, and it all starts with understanding what the goals are. Remembering that there are three main ways that CFF-CBT combined with medication will help stabilize your child's mood and improve overall functioning can give you the confidence to stick with the program when you feel overwhelmed and start to wonder whether anything is really working:

1. **Symptom control:** First, at a symptom level, CFF-CBT aims to reduce excitability, elated mood, depression, and irritability primarily through the use of medication and establishing a routine.

2. **Emotional modulation (as informed by research on brain function):** At a biological–brain level, CFF-CBT is designed to reduce emotional overreactivity. Our brain studies have shown that bipolar children cannot think clearly if they are drenched in negative emotions. The area of the brain that appraises emotions in the first instance is called the amygdala, an almond-shaped organ. Our studies of bipolar youth showed excessive activity in the amygdala in response to negative stimuli, with the ventrolateral prefrontal cortex being inefficient in modulating the amygdala. The dorsolateral part of the prefrontal cortex in the brain, which helps us strategize and think, appeared to underfunction whenever the amygdala was overactive. While this model is simplified, especially given the multitude of other complex connections, it is highly informative and forms the basis for our treatment model. We think that medication and RAINBOW therapy will reverse this affect dysregulation and stabilize mood (see the diagram of the brain on the facing page).

These children are disturbed too easily when exposed to criticism or perceived criticism. Therefore, based on our studies of blood flow changes in the presence of negative emotions in these children, we specifically designed empathy-based RAINBOW therapy (CFF-CBT) to work with the philosophy of reducing any negativity around them. The goal is to create a nurturing, positive environment, reducing perceived threats and decreasing chances for provocation, to help them think clearly and solve problems more easily.

Note, too, that the frontal systems of the brain are connected to the basal ganglia at the subcortical regions, or lower parts of the brain. The involvement of the fronto-striatal system appears to underlie cognitive problems such as inattention and inhibition. For now, I will not go into

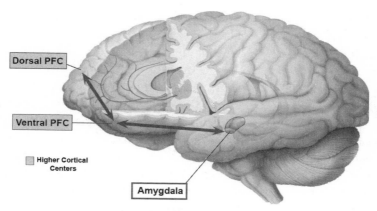

The fronto-limbic system.

too much detail, other than to say that several circuits are involved, the fronto-limbic circuit being a major one that explains affect dysregulation.

Elements of self-psychology are helpful here, too. In the self-psychology model, you serve as a mirror and source of praise and validation to help your child see herself more positively. In other words, you feed her sense of self—those inner feelings of goodness—by showing that you value her. That is why I think the old saying "Spare the rod and spoil the child" should be replaced with "Spare the love and spoil the child." The approach seeks to improve family interactions, decrease conflict in the home, and limit the stressors that can trigger mood fluctuations. Thus, the brain model of bipolar children leads us also to move away from implementing negative consequences. "You are grounded!" is a phrase we want to avoid as much as possible. Note that this is a radical change from implementing the negative consequences of behavior therapy.

3. **Family functioning and parents as coaches:** CFF-CBT focuses on family relationships, on understanding and supporting the family as a whole unit. It has been my observation that the short- and long-term success of treatment depends strongly on the leadership of parents and the cooperation of other members of the family. It's not hard to see that the whole family is affected by the presence of the bipolar child, and, thus, the entire family plays a role in management of the disorder; the onus is especially on parents receiving cognitive therapy for themselves and learning to apply the techniques at the same time to their bipolar child.

CFF-CBT can help parents and other family members understand the illness and the best ways to manage it, and, therefore, be better able to help their child.

Within this context, cognitive strategies are used to enhance positive thinking, based on the idea that many depressed people have a negative or pessimistic thinking process that encourages feelings of helplessness and hopelessness. The goal of therapy is to help the bipolar child reframe her outlook so she can more effectively cope with life's inevitable challenges and disappointments. When bad things happen, the bipolar child might think she is to blame and/or is unusually unlucky and begin to expect the worst all the time. CFF-CBT helps the child develop a more realistic view of the world, recognize the possibilities for positive outcomes, learn to negotiate inevitable barriers in life, and thereby decrease the tendency for depression and anxiety. Thus, you as the parent become a coach for your child. You learn to model the skills you learn for your child. You will involve your other children, so that they can understand and empathize with the struggles of the affected child. Read on and discover how to bring this philosophy into your family's life.

Making the Most of Your Child's Treatment: A New Philosophy

In Chapters 5 and 6, I will describe this approach in detail and specifically explain how you can incorporate it into your family's daily life. But before we get into the nitty-gritty details, I want to share some "therapeutic pearls" that I have gleaned from long experience treating bipolar disorder in children. These basic concepts reflect a philosophy and mindset that can make all the difference when you are dealing with the complex and turbulent world of childhood bipolar disorder. They reflect an orientation that will help you, the parent, help your child, yourself, and the rest of your family on the road to success:

1. **Take the pressure off:** There is so much pressure in American or any affluent, urban society to achieve and make sure our children keep up with their peers. But children with bipolar disorder cannot maintain the pace their parents would like or even that the children themselves would prefer. Don't be driven by the pack; set your own pace! Tell yourself your

story is yours. Appreciate your child's unique strengths, accept his weaknesses, and try not to worry about how he compares to other children. Focus on what he can do now, and let go of expectations for the future. Reinforce the best characteristics and attitudes of your child, and gently teach him to develop his strengths in the course of daily events. "Teaching by influence"—by being flexible, compassionate, and persistent—will prove invaluable.

2. **Target a few things and keep at it:** It is extremely difficult to target every single negative behavior that your child may display. It's better to pick a few important issues and make a consistent, gentle effort to correct them. For instance, if the problem is slamming doors and kicking, provide a gentle correction every single time your child deviates from your expectations. Consistent, gentle repetition will create an "inner voice of conscience" that helps ingrain a new habit of being cooperative. You may think, "Oh no, the mania is coming back," but, even with mood-moderating medications, oppositional behavior and reactivity is a problem that takes time to subside. If you engage in constant criticism to address this problem, your child is likely to tune you out. Parents often say, "I tried, and it goes in one ear and out the other." In my experience, if parents focus on one thing at a time, the lesson eventually sinks in. In fact, I've seen this work many times with the most recalcitrant children. Consistent commitment and firmness from parents really pay off!

3. **Cultivate your child's "islands of competence":** It is important to identify and cultivate one shining quality that your bipolar child can own. For example, Sarah is a fantastic artist. She has a natural flair and draws the most beautiful pictures you could imagine. I could not resist the temptation to ask her if I could frame one of her pictures for my office. She could be a future Van Gogh! Nurturing these extraordinary qualities could change Sarah's life, rather than her parents pressuring her to excel in mathematics, which drives her to tears every single time. Children (and adults, for that matter) have "islands of competence," even brilliance. They know what they are good at. Help them recognize that no one is good at everything. **Let them build on their islands of competence, and you will see the small islands slowly join together to build self-confidence and promote self-esteem.**

4. **Get respect by giving it:** Bipolar children's lack of emotional control can result in pretty disrespectful behavior at times, and it's up to parents to insist that they adhere to some basic courtesies. One of the best ways to get your child to show respect is to demonstrate it by displaying

compassion and respect for him and the other people in your lives, including your spouse and friends, your child's grandparents, and other relatives. These days, families tend to be separated by distance and time, coming together only for holidays and special occasions. Use these get-togethers as opportunities to teach your child to care about and respect his family and appreciate his roots. Encourage elders to share family history and honor them with a special place at the dining table. Invite them to join you and your child at church, on a dinner outing, or for a dance recital or sporting event. This instantly shows how much you value these relationships and helps your child internalize family values. Caring for elders and other family members will also help your child take the focus off his own feelings and frustrations and place a higher priority on the feelings of others—helping him modulate his feelings and behavior based on the value system that is slowly internalized. Requiring your bipolar child to say please and thank you as often as possible will help him get along better socially. Gentle repetition will be needed to make the lesson stick. Remember always to treat your child like you would a well-liked next-door neighbor. You may wonder, "Why should I be behaving in a formal way to my own child?" but this technique will help moderate the intensity generated between you and your bipolar child.

5. **Take back control:** Does your bipolar child grab the remote control, scowl, and scream at you when you ask for it back? Does she constantly contradict you? Does she act like she is queen of the house? Does she verbally attack you at home or lash out in public, no matter who's watching? This is not a result of your "spoiling" her, as some uninformed observers might suggest, but a reflection of the extreme irritability and reactivity that accompanies bipolar disorder. Unfortunately, because your bipolar child can be so *out of control*, she ends up *controlling you*. You end up accommodating her and yielding to her moods in order to keep the peace at home and to protect your marriage and your other children. You are not a wimp but a person caught in the middle, trying to manage a difficult child while maintaining a livable home. To live with this difficult situation, *you must take back control*—that is, be the boss, assert your power as the parent, and set appropriate limits for your bipolar child. Knowing that there are limits and that parents are going to uphold them actually gives children a sense of security. I recognize that this is definitely harder to do with bipolar children—they will push you to the max—but it is important to make your expectations clear and stand your ground. I will talk more about this in later chapters, but suffice it to say here that taking

back control, nicely, is a critical strategy for managing bipolar disorder on a daily basis. Here's one way to think about it: "I can stay powerful without engaging in verbal fights to prove my superiority. I can be gentle, firm, and powerful." An important point to remember here is that if you raise your voice, your child may yell back, and then all hell will break loose. One smart way to attain control is to withdraw and stop talking to the child, being serious and dignified. Your child will realize her mistakes and plead guilty sooner or later. You can then say that you are concerned about her behavior and will discuss the issue later, when you both cool down.

6. **Sticks and stones . . . :** You have no doubt heard your child call you "stupid" or an "idiot" or "moron" more than once, and it's hard not to react to it, feel embarrassed about it, or take it to heart. I counsel parents not to invest a lot of energy in these words. "I keep remembering it is the bipolar talking," said one mother, " not the child, and try as often as I can to speak with firmness, but loving kindness: 'This behavior is not acceptable, and we love you and will help you learn to control it; when we see you cannot control yourself, we will help you.'" Bipolar children can have "diarrhea of the mouth," and they frequently can't control what comes out of their mouths. It is best to stay detached in the face of these tirades. Again, it is a matter of not letting it control you. It works best to stay calm, explain that these words are disrespectful, and withdraw for a few minutes or hours, as I said above, to convey your displeasure. I'm not suggesting giving them the cold shoulder, but send the message that you are not willing to be treated like that. By the time you calm down, your child will also come around to apologizing or at least backing down to a degree. Don't hold a grudge; let it roll off you "like water off a duck's back" and move on! Start fresh every single time. You have to swallow some unsavory stuff, and I bet you can do it well.

7. **Follow through:** When you give your child a directive, he needs to know that you mean business. Be committed to following through and leave no room for negotiations or pushing the boundaries. Gentle but unequivocal guidance from you will teach your child to reach your mutual goals. If there's a huge tantrum, explosion, and rage, give it some time to run its course. "We know when Joe's mood is escalating, and we either try to redirect or give him space to pull himself together," Joe's mother says. "Talking calmly (which is not always easy) and telling him to go to his room for a little bit and listen to his music sometimes helps." Of course, there are times you will fail and things hit the ceiling. Pick up the threads

again at the next opportunity. You can always go through what happened when your child is in a good mood and have a positive, constructive talk about what happened and how you would have preferred she behave. That way you end up giving the child the message of what is expected and reasonable.

Keep in mind before you start:

- Keep the pressure low: Set your own pace, be flexible, and let go of expectations.
- Focus on one or two things at a time: Starting out with fewer goals will help you stick with them.
- Cultivate your child's islands of competence: Know where she shines and help her build self-esteem by promoting what she's good at.
- Model respect: Live by your family's values and you'll benefit from the golden rule.
- Remember that you're in charge: Benevolent authority will help keep bipolar disorder from ruling your life.
- Don't take it personally: You can convey your disapproval of your child's verbal disrespect without holding a grudge. Start fresh and move on after that!
- Follow through: You may not be able to get through to your child in the middle of a rage or even right after, but you can keep stressing behavior standards in calmer moments.

For many of you, trying to use these principles in your day-to-day life will feel like a tall order, particularly if you and your child are still struggling to get the right diagnosis or find the right treatment program. But I assure you that you *can* cultivate the necessary skills to handle many challenging situations if you approach them with the right mindset and support. In Chapter 7, I will expand more on how to hone your parenting skills to apply these principles and become your child's best advocate. Yes, you are the secret weapon in the battle against childhood bipolar disorder, and I want to give you all the equipment and support you need to succeed.

Finally, many of the same principles can help with the management of bipolar disorder at home, school, and other outside activities, as I will discuss in depth in Part III. Now, let's turn to the role medication and mood management play in treating bipolar disorder in children.

FIVE

Managing Your Child's Moods with Medication

"Her moods are mostly stable with the combo of meds she is now on—this is the first stability she's seen since her diagnosis. The right meds can be amazing!"

Medication plays a critical role in treating children with bipolar disorder. Without the mood-stabilizing effect of medication, it is difficult for psychotherapy and behavior management interventions to take full effect. This is particularly true if there are comorbid conditions or multiple symptoms. Parents whose children have received the appropriate medication will swear by its ability to moderate their children's moods and open the door to therapy. I also get professional satisfaction watching medications work their magic. They are the most powerful tools I have in my bag of tricks, but I also realize that I have the responsibility to use them carefully.

It is important to understand that medication isn't the be-all and end-all for some bipolar children. Even when they do respond, there is still a lot of trial and error involved. Children are often treated with multiple medications, inadvertently in partial or excessive doses. These medications frequently are not given an adequate trial, and new ones are layered on, making it unclear which medication is working. In fact, even in research studies that are supposed to guide treatment, often the trial periods are too short and investigators have not always been able to recruit or maintain patients in the studies because of the complex nature of the disorder. Undoubtedly, as our understanding of the disorder and its impact on the child's developing brain and physiology advances, studies will become more rigorous and we will improve our ability to find the right treatment more quickly.

We recently tested a medication algorithm (a step-by-step model for trying different medications based on the child's symptoms and responses until the best fit is found) with a group of children with bipolar disorder associated with our program. We closely monitored the patients for 18 months, and if new symptoms emerged, worsened, or there was a poor response, we made strategic medication changes according to the algorithm. At the end of the study, there were significant differences between the algorithm group and the treatment-as-usual group, with the children following the algorithm showing greater symptom reduction and better overall functioning. However, the response rate was only 68%. These results suggest that although medication management of bipolar disorder is an ongoing process requiring careful adjustment and follow-up, as many as 30% of patients may not respond to medication by itself.

The other problem is that things change rapidly, and a medication, combination of medications, or dosage that worked one day may not work another. "We try again and again and again to find *something* that will work, and just when we find some improvement, my son *grows* or develops tolerance and we are back at square one," said one mother, lamenting a somewhat unavoidable problem. That's why close monitoring of your child's mood is so important, along with maintaining good communication with your doctor about how your child is responding to a particular course of therapy. In addition, the CFF-CBT approach that I introduced in Chapter 4 will help you, your child, and the rest of your family work together in ways that will directly or indirectly support your child's medication treatment so that the bipolar child gets the most improvement possible from the medicine. You'll read in more detail about how this works in Chapter 6.

Common Medication Dilemmas

Medication management of bipolar disorder can be tricky. In some ways it is still as much an art as a science.

Anticipating Trial and Error

It can take a lot of trial and error to find the combination that's right for your child. One family went through three different doctors, who prescribed everything from Haldol (haloperidol) to Prozac (fluoxetine) to lithium, until they found the right combination of medications that worked for their son. Doctors who treat this disorder must rely on the available literature, their real-world experience, and feedback from you and your child about how a particular medication or combination of medications is working. That's why it's so important that you have a good rapport with your doctor and that you try to keep good records on mood states, physical reactions, and other data needed to make informed prescribing decisions. *A history of medications, doses, and your child's response to them is the single most valuable collection of information you can keep to show your doctor (see Appendices D and E for logs).*

Weighing the Risks

Parents sometimes are afraid to try certain drugs because they read about frightening side effects on the Internet or hear about them in the news. A classic example is the recent controversy about suicidal thoughts and behaviors by children and adolescents using selective serotonin reuptake inhibitors (SSRIs), discussed later in this chapter. Similarly, you might read that lithium can affect the kidneys or that atypical antipsychotics can cause diabetes. The information provided by pharmaceutical companies, which must include every conceivable adverse reaction and risk, also can be pretty off-putting. These risks are real, but the risks of untreated bipolar disorder can be significantly greater, and you need to discuss your concerns with your clinician, who can filter the more serious or common side effects from the plethora of possible side effects. The most relevant side effects of each medication are listed in my *Handbook of Psychopharmacotherapy* (see the Resources).

Uninformed Is Unarmed

When you discuss medication options with your doctor, take along a list of your concerns and go over them one by one. Your doctor should be able to explain the expected benefits and warn you of any risks based on clinical evidence and experience, but you shouldn't get overly worried about every potential problem. Of course, it's helpful to keep the information on the drug with you in case an obscure symptom develops. That way you can report it and see if it is medication-related, a symptom of the illness, or due to another cause, then make appropriate adjustments.

**Questions to Ask Your Child's Doctor
about Medications**

It's important to discuss the following questions with your child's provider
when any medication is being considered:

- How does the medication work?
- Have studies been done on the medication?
- Which tests need to be done before my child starts the medication?
- How soon will I see improvement?
- What will be the signs of improvement?
- How often will my child have to take the medication?
- How and under what circumstances will the decision be made to stop
  it?
- What are the negative side effects of the medication?
- What will happen if my child doesn't take it?
- How do we handle a missed dose?

Keeping Track of What *Didn't* Work

By the same token, be sure to inform the doctor of any bad experiences
your child has had with a particular medication. Often, children with
bipolar disorder have seen multiple doctors and tried many approaches
before they are diagnosed. Your child may have been misdiagnosed as having simple ADHD or depression and, thus, been put on stimulants or antidepressants, with predictably negative consequences. Or your child may
have been diagnosed correctly, but had a negative experience with one of
the typical mainline medications. Sometimes a doctor who isn't trained in
pediatric bipolar disorder or isn't up on the latest research or critically
important scientific developments will suggest trying a drug that you
know from experience is harmful to your child. When planning your
child's medication treatment, the doctor should take a history of which
medications worsened the child's condition in the past, which were ineffective, and which were somewhat useful or helpful for a period of time.

Remember that you have the right to refuse a treatment for your
child when you know it has been ineffective or damaging. "You have to
remember that you are the expert on your child—don't let anyone else
tell you otherwise," said one father. The same parent, however, uttered an

important caution that I echo: "You must educate yourself and be sure that you glean all the necessary information about the resources available and keep looking." This means that you should never shy away from working with your doctor; feel free to share information on medications you've gathered, but take whatever care you can to ensure that it's from up-to-date, scientifically reliable sources and always present it respectfully to the doctor, especially if a physician recommends an antidepressant and you know from past experience that your child is likely to have a strong negative reaction to it. A well-trained physician will respect your experience and listen to your story, more so if you have kept good documentation about what happened with a medication in the past. I'll talk more about acting as an advocate for your child in Chapter 7.

Occasionally, I have parents come to me with no record of which medications have been tried, but this does not present an insurmountable obstacle to treatment. In fact, sometimes it gives me a clean slate from which to develop the ideal medication regime. Parents are sometimes able to rattle off a list of previous medications, but it may not preclude me from trying some of them again—previous trials may not have been at the optimal dose or in the optimal combination, or things may have changed significantly since the medication was tried. As long as your doctor is using a careful step-by-step process and closely monitoring the results, it doesn't hurt to try various medications in a logical order.

Must Medications Have FDA Approval for Children?

The United States Food and Drug Administration (FDA) performs an important oversight function by ensuring that medications are tested for both safety and effectiveness, usually through large clinical trials involving many adult volunteers. With the exception of lithium (age 12 and above) and risperidone (Risperdal) (age 10 and above), most of the medications used to treat childhood bipolar disorder are not FDA approved for this use. It is likely that other medications may get approval in the course of time as drug companies are encouraged by the FDA to conduct pediatric trials. Prescribing drugs not approved for pediatric use is not necessarily harmful or risky, although all medications should be tried under the close supervision of a qualified physician. If you have concerns about the use of a particular medication for your child, be sure to discuss them with your physician to determine why she thinks it is a good choice for your child.

Medication Reality Check

Keep these three caveats in mind to maintain a realistic outlook on your child's medication treatment:

1. This is a marathon, not a sprint. There are very few overnight miracles. This is potentially a long haul in which symptoms can occur at random and new illness cycles can start unpredictably. Also, it takes time for some medications to build up in the bloodstream before they have an effect. It's a step-by-step process, tailored to every child's illness and history of medication response, and varies a lot by individual. One of my own studies of preschool-onset bipolar patients showed that symptoms don't start to stabilize until after approximately 4–6 months of medication. This coincides with our clinical experience, in which it is common for families to spread their visits to once every 3 months after the initial follow-up period once the child's moods are stabilized.

2. Larger doses are not always better. It may seem obvious to suggest that your child's doctor up the dosage if a medication isn't having the desired effect, but there is an optimal dose for each medication, and more isn't always better. Be alert for prescriptions for a high dose of risperidone; research in my own clinic suggests that 1 to 2 mg is optimal (the average is around 1 mg if your child is an outpatient). Similarly, high doses of mixed amphetamine salts (Adderall XR) or methylphenidate (Ritalin) often cause serious problems, worsen symptoms, or even cause psychosis due to high dopamine levels. Underdosing is also a problem, mainly because it delays the mood stabilization that the medications are supposed to produce. We have seen children enter our clinic taking 150- or 300-mg doses of oxcarbazepine (Trileptal), way below the therapeutic window, so this is one to watch for.

3. Medications shouldn't be changed precipitously, but again, if they are harmful, we may need to stop them quickly. At our clinic we frequently hear complaints from parents that "Our doctor changes medications too quickly" or "Our doctor did not stop the medication when it was doing more harm than good." As I said above, sticking with a medication through a complete trial is important, especially if there is at least partial response. At the same time, if symptoms get worse, the doctor needs to stop the medication quickly, sometimes immediately instead of through a slow withdrawal. I normally call for knocking off one pill every other day, whatever the medication may be, at varying strengths, but this is something that must be sorted out with your own doctor. I would be ready to move on to another medication when there is absolutely **no response** in 2 weeks in the case of antipsychotics or stimulants, although this rule does not apply for mood stabilizers that can take longer to begin working. Even small signs of calming down in your child represent a partial response and probably mean you should stick with the medication.

What Are Our Medication Choices?

There are four basic types of medications your child's doctor may prescribe:

- Mood stabilizers
- Second-generation antipsychotics
- Antidepressants
- "Adjunctive" medications used to treat bipolar symptoms, comorbid conditions, and side effects

The goals of medication management are to establish the greatest level of mood stabilization, to keep your child in the "safe" middle zone (which I will explain further in Chapter 6). But because of the variability of bipolar disorder and your child's changing physiology, very often a particular drug will work partially or only for a period of time, necessitating a change in regimen. Where your doctor starts and what she ultimately prescribes will depend on your child's mood state and his response to a trial of a particular medication.

You'll find more details on commonly prescribed medications in Appendix F, along with a suggested reading list in the Resources that includes a book I wrote with Dr. Philip Janicak called *Handbook of Psychopharmacotherapy*. This will serve as a handy reference when you need to remind yourself of important facts about your child's medications, but remember that your child's doctor should be your primary source of information and insight. As I tell families: "I went to medical school to be trained in all of it for you. I will do the worrying and try to do my best. Ask me questions if you have doubts. But don't put the burden of figuring this all out on your shoulders." What I'm saying is that we'll work together to do the best for your child, and I'll count on you to report what you observe in her. No doctor should leave you feeling as if you have to worry about every single detail of your child's treatment. That is your doctor's job. If your questions aren't being answered sufficiently, ask again.

Your doctor may not inform you of all possible side effects of a medication so as not to alarm you needlessly. Generally, you only need to be aware of the most common or potentially serious side effects. However, if you notice anything unusual, be prepared to mention it immediately to your doctor. You can use the Pediatric Side Effects Checklist (P-SEC) in Appendix E to help keep track of your child's reactions.

In addition to traditional medications, alternative therapies and "biologic agents" such as omega-3 fatty acids, choline, inositol, and micronutrients or megavitamins are increasingly being proposed for treating bipolar disorder in children. I will talk about what we know about the value of these therapies and the associated realities along with the pros and cons of using these a little later in this chapter.

Which Medications Should Be Stopped

• *Ineffective medications:* After a 2-week trial (or longer for medications that take longer to show effects), the child should be reasonably quickly weaned off anything that has absolutely no positive effect, though the time for tapering is highly variable depending on the situation.

• *Antidepressants:* Despite compelling evidence that antidepressants worsen bipolar symptoms either by switching those who take them to mania or by worsening mania, children are still being treated with substantial doses. Because children with the disorder generally experience a combination of depression, anxiety, and restlessness, many physicians tune in to depressive symptoms at the cost of making mania worse. Therefore, antidepressants, in particular SSRIs such as sertraline (Zoloft), fluoxetine (Prozac), escitalopram (Lexapro), or bupropion (Wellbutrin) should be discontinued. (From here on, I will try to use trade names, as most parents are familiar with those names; you can find the generic names in Appendix F. Readers from outside the United States can cross-refer to decode the local drugs based on this list.)

• *Stimulants:* Mood stabilization is the first priority, so any stimulants your child is taking to control symptoms of ADHD should be discontinued until his or her moods are stabilized. If it looks like stimulants are helping despite their impact on your child's mood, the doctor may choose to continue the stimulants but should do so at the lowest possible doses and in long-acting form, while quickly adding a mood stabilizer before the child's mood spirals into mania or mania mixed with depression.

First Treatment Choices

Whether your child is showing symptoms of mania or depression, the first treatment of choice for bipolar children continues to be a mood stabilizer such as lithium or Depakote (divalproex) due to their established track record of preventive properties (mainly based on studies of adult bipolar disorder); however, lithium or Depakote may not always be effective and/ or will be slow to act. Recent unpublished industry data on Depakote has been disappointing in children, although some published non-industry-initiated trials report divided results. I often think of prescribing Lamictal (lamotrigine) as the first choice if depressive symptoms are mixed with mania. It takes a while to work, as you dose this drug rather slowly to begin with, in order to avoid rash that could be life-threatening but is extremely rare when the medication is dosed appropriately. Consequently, second-generation antipsychotics (SGAs) such as Risperdal and Abilify (aripiprazole) are rapidly finding their place either as the only medication (in emergency situations where stabilizing mania is a priority) or in combination with a mood stabilizer. My own research shows that SGAs alone may be effective when irritability is prominent and demands a faster response not possible with first-line mood stabilizers.

A Proven Step-by-Step Approach to Medications

As I mentioned in the Introduction, the following model resulted in 68% of the children and adolescents treated in my clinic being stabilized from illness over an 18-month period:

1. Stopping antidepressants or other mismatched medications that the child is currently taking (see the list of medications that should be stopped on page 250).
2. Treating with mood stabilizers or antipsychotics together or alone (see pages 90–93 for information on first-line medication choices and combination therapy).
3. Treating comorbid conditions after mood stabilization is achieved (see the discussion on page 95).
4. Problem-solving further to address unresolved symptoms and adverse events.

A Close-Up of How I Prescribe Medications

On pages 100 and 101 you'll read about the medication trials of a couple of children that I consider representative of what a lot of children will experience on their way to managing their moods through medication. Here, I want to give you a closer look at the medications I have found most effective and how I prescribe them—where I've found them most useful, starting doses and incremental increases I use during a medication trial, the forms in which the drug is available, side effects typically encountered and how I address them, and other factors involved in administering the medication that you should be aware of. I hope this will give you a very good grasp of what you might expect when your child begins treatment.

What do I consider at the start? First, to prescribe medication, every doctor thinks about the dose appropriate for the particular weight and age of the child. For easy reference to weight, I divide children into three groups: those age 8 and under, those in middle childhood (between age 9 and 12), and teenagers. Consider which of the three groups your child falls into as you read about the following medications.

Second, remember that there is no rule of thumb in prescribing any of these medications. **Every child tolerates and responds very differently to these medications.**

Third, I almost always prescribe mood stabilizers and stimulants in long-acting form or prescribe all medications to be taken at night. This strategy minimizes the hassle of taking medications at multiple times and takes advantage of their sedative properties. Keep in mind throughout the following discussion that I am talking about dosages geared to children being treated as outpatients, living in a normal home setting. The children I see on my regular rounds in our university's inpatient facility are very sick and often somewhat heavyset, and they require on average at least a third of a dose higher than what I am suggesting here.

Finally, I have excluded medications that are either peripheral to the management of children with bipolar disorder, such as Clonidine, or not that useful, such as Neurontin (gabapentin).

As I've said throughout this book, after stopping certain medications the child may already be taking, my first goal is to stabilize his moods. **The following are the mood stabilizers I prescribe, in order of preference:**

Lithium

Lithium is a classic mood stabilizer considered to be neuroprotective and helpful in stabilizing mood. By "neuroprotection," I mean that this medication is known to reduce nerve cell death and help in sprouting new nerve cells. In fact, I describe this medication to families as really solid. What I mean by that is that children don't develop quick tolerance to it once it starts working, especially along with some other atypical anti-psychotic medication, and persistence with a trial of several weeks generally pays off.

The downside? It takes time for lithium to start working. You have to wait at least 2 months, sometimes even 4, before it begins to show its muscles. Meanwhile, your child will have to have several lab tests to determine her blood levels of lithium, which will help the doctor determine the appropriate dosage. Blood levels could be anywhere from 0.6 to 1.3 mEq/L, with a maintenance dose blood level tending to be below 1 mEq/L mmols/L. Lab tests should check not just for serum levels but also for hypothyroidism and kidney function.

Lithium comes in 150- or 300-mg tablets, so think of increments in those round figures when you think of how dosages break down for kids of different ages. Usually with very young children I would start lithium at 150 mg twice a day and increase it to 300 mg twice a day. For kids in middle childhood, I go up to 900 to 1,200 mg. Teenagers tolerate up to 1,800–2,000 mg—however, I am guided more by the response, serum level, and tolerability. The liquid lithium citrate is available if your child cannot take the tablets.

A typical side effect to be aware of is enuresis, especially bedwetting. Your child may feel thirsty when taking lithium, so don't stop him from drinking water even if bedwetting becomes a problem.

Trileptal

Trileptal is my next favorite medication, despite the fact that a study published shortly before this book went to press indicated it is only as good as taking a placebo, or sugar pill. This drug, in my experience of working with scores of youngsters, works very well for aggression in pediatric bipolar disorder, and, therefore, I think of it as the "Risperdal among mood stabilizers" given its similar effectiveness in reducing aggression. (As a clinician/scientist, I am forced to make careful judgments weighing research evidence against my own solid experience as a clinician. At times, I may choose medication based on the intricate symptom profile of bipolar kids rather than just the broad umbrella of diagnosis. This is where science as it stands now cannot always do justice to real-life practice.) When Trileptal became available, I stopped using its brother compound, Tegretol (carbamazepine), as much, as Trileptal has fewer side effects and has the advantage of not requiring blood tests. It is a good idea to check for reduction in sodium levels when a child is taking Trileptal, as it is a known, although infrequent, side effect of this medication.

I would prescribe this medication at 150 mg twice a day in very young children, increasing to 600 mg and then 900 mg for a school-age child, and 900–1,200 mg in teenagers. Trileptal (and Tegretol) are prescribed in divided doses to be given twice a day given the nature of their half-lives in the body.

Very rarely, rash and double vision have been noted in children taking Trileptal. Both side effects are harmless, but I stop the medication if there is rash and reduce the dose if there is double vision.

Depakote

Depakote also continues to be an important choice as a mood stabilizer; however, there are severe gastrointestinal side effects, weight gain, and sedation that can make it difficult to tolerate. Kids can get excitable after taking Depakote for a short period, but, if it works, it does a good job of reducing excitability and stabilizing mood. Be aware that blood levels, liver function tests, and complete blood count need to be monitored on a regular basis.

I would prescribe this at 125 mg twice a day in very young children, going up to 250 mg twice a day, and gradually increasing to 1,000 or 1,250 mg depending on the age of the child. In very high doses of approximately 1,200 mg, both Trileptal and Depakote show their efficacy within 2–3 weeks. Teens, especially heavyset individuals or those who metabolize faster, may require higher doses of up to 1,500–2,000 mg. Depakote comes in once-a-day slow-release form, and I tend to prescribe only the nighttime dose. This drug increases the dose of Lamictal by slowing its metabolism and may cause rash as blood Lamictal levels may inadvertently go up. So, I tend to be extra cautious and avoid prescribing these two drugs together—although half the normal dose of Depakote is considered by some doctors as appropriate while managing the combined regime.

Lamictal

Lamictal is a medication I use to a great degree for type II bipolar disorder with predominant depression. It's almost used as an antidepressant in bipolar children, sometimes by itself during the maintenance phase or, more commonly, in combination with antipsychotics and rarely in combination with lithium. When it works, it is really miraculous how children recover from depression and associated mixed symptoms of bipolarity. Remember, though, that this drug does not necessarily work by itself in the acute stage.

The most important thing to remember with this medication is that it needs to be increased very slowly, or there is a risk of a serious rash. If introduced very slowly, rash is very rare, and, even if it occurs, it tends to be a benign rash that can easily be taken care of with the use of cortisol or an oral antihistamine that any family practitioner or psychiatrist can prescribe. Children develop fever and need to be kept out of school, and the rash goes away in most instances in 5–6 days.

I usually start at a low dose of 12.5 mg per day and increase it by 12.5 mg every week until I reach up to 200 mg. Usually children of any age do not tolerate the drug over 200 mg and tend to get agitated. In younger children, I would stop the dosing at 150 mg but go up to 200 mg in older children. Like Trileptal, Lamictal is prescribed in divided doses to be given twice a day given the nature of its half-life in the body. No major blood tests are necessary for this drug.

Topamax

Topamax (topiramate) is a drug that I prescribe very rarely these days, mainly as an adjuvant at around 100 mg. Along with a mood stabilizer or another antipsychotic, I use it to tone down weight gain, but the results are often mediocre at best.

As to the second-generation antipsychotics (SGAs) or neuroleptic medications, they are quick to act and are much more efficacious in treating acute states than even mood stabilizers. Very often, I go for the SGAs before I add a mood stabilizer to get the symptoms under control. There are times when I would not want to prescribe a mood stabilizer because of lethargy, sedation, and the need for regular blood tests to monitor lipid levels. SGAs generally start working within 1 week, and you and the doctor should be able to tell if one is effective within 2 weeks before you make any alteration. With any SGA, it is extremely important to dose gingerly. High doses are not necessarily going to be helpful and will, in fact, hinder progress. Again, combining these medications and offering optimal doses is a delicate balancing act.

Risperdal

What I like about this SGA is its efficacy for aggression, irritability, mania, and the full spectrum of manic symptoms. The main worries with this medication are weight gain, extrapyramidal side effects (uncomfortable and frightening affects such as eyes rolling backward, stiff jaw and arm muscles, and tremors), and prolactin elevation (which may result in breast enlargement and secretions or no overt clinical signs; as we do not know of the long-term effects of this rise, we recommend caution). You would start with 0.25 mg twice a day of Risperdal, increasing it to 0.5 mg twice a day. Regardless of age, I never go beyond 2 mg in the regular outpatient setting for young children. If it's not working at 2 mg, I would rather shift to another medication than increase it to a higher dose.

Seroquel

Seroquel (quetiapine) is my other choice when children are either depressed or somewhat anxious, especially those who need sleep at night. I prescribe Seroquel at 200 mg at nighttime. In general, for efficacy, I go anywhere from 50 mg, especially as an adjuvant, to a 500-mg dose. What is interesting about this medication is that there is a wide range of safety with no major side effects other than perhaps sedation and weight gain. Lipid levels need to be monitored on a regular basis. This is the one medication that I do not hesitate to prescribe as an adjuvant to other antipsychotics (I almost never give two SGAs together) for sleep problems.

Abilify

Abilify is prescribed in doses between 2.5 mg in very young children and an average of 10 mg for middle childhood. This is a great drug for psychosis. Extrapyramidal side effects (described above) are a huge issue when taking this medication, so I often prescribe Cogentin (benztropine) at 1 mg a day with it, especially if I think that this particular child is sensitive to any type of medication. Nausea and vomiting are common side effects, especially at the initiation of this drug.

Geodon

Geodon (ziprasidone) is the other medication that is my favorite when I would like to focus on reducing weight gain for those who are extremely self-conscious or affected by other mood stabilizers in terms of weight gain. This medication is also known to work well for mixed or depressive states. Extrapyramidal side effects are the major worry with this medication, and I do not hesitate to prescribe Cogentin alongside it. Children generally do not tolerate very high doses, unlike adults, which means it's often difficult to get to an optimal efficacious dose. As specified, it is prescribed at 20 mg twice a day, increasing to 20 mg A.M. and 40 mg P.M. to up to 100 mg on average. Again, all of these doses can be pushed a little higher in teenagers who are heavyset or extremely disruptive.

Zyprexa

Zyprexa (olanzapine) is a drug that I rarely prescribe because of severe weight gain in children. Again, although some children do well on this medication (it's extremely efficacious), lipids need to be monitored very carefully.

Clozaril

Clozaril (clozapine) can be useful in treatment-resistant cases, but the regular blood draws to check white blood cell count make it low on my list, and I have to confess that I have not prescribed this drug to many children, although I found it very useful when I used it. Especially in chronic bipolar disorder with negative symptoms and psychosis, I noted several patients get their lives back to a great degree!

Psychostimulants

Psychostimulants are often used to treat the neurocognitive symptoms of poor attention span and working memory problems in these children and, to some extent, to improve their executive functioning (the ability to control and deliberately apply mental skills). One important thing to remember, however, is that there is no role for short-acting stimulants at the current time. The long-acting form, which lasts about 12 hours, can be used in the morning as a single dose. Where there is a need, a small amount of immediate-release stimulant (a short-acting drug that lasts anywhere from 4 to 6 hours) can be used at 3:00 or 4:00 P.M. (the latest time that it should be used) so the child can do homework. There are several ice hockey goalies in my practice, and many times parents have pushed me to give Adderall at 6:00 P.M. so they can focus on evening games, but I am leery about doing this.

Usually, I also worry about the upper limit of these stimulants, as children walk in my door with very high doses of stimulants and my immediate job is to reduce them to the optimal level or stop them. Stimulants can make bipolar children pretty manic at very high doses without another adjuvant medication on board. *I would never recommend Adderall XR being prescribed beyond 40 mg, Ritalin over 60 mg, or Concerta (methylphenidate) over 54 mg.* Of course, Strattera (atomoxetine) does not work like a stimulant; it's a different type of medication that needs to be given at nighttime, and usually the highest dose is no more than 120 mg in young children and 160 mg in teenagers.

With regard to anxiety and depression, I resist prescribing for them. The type of child who cries out for a medication to treat anxiety or depression is the one who curls up in a fetal position, who tends to be severely anxious, has severe panic attacks, can't go to school or do anything, worries constantly, and gets agitated and unable to cope. Once I know that an antipsychotic or mood stabilizer is on board, I carefully prescribe a very small dose of an antidepressant to these kids, such as 10 mg of Lexapro or an equivalent of this dose of any SSRI, *but followed very carefully. If deterioration in terms of agitation, aggressiveness, irritability, silliness, giggling, and euphoria increases within a week, this medication needs to be stopped.*

A Typical Medication Trial for Mood Stabilization

Four to 6 weeks at therapeutic blood levels (blood levels apply to some but not all mood stabilizers but not to antipsychotics) and/or an adequate dose (8 weeks of treatment may be required for some drugs, such as lithium) of:

1. Lithium or Depakote
2. Lamictal for mixed depression and mania
3. Second-generation antipsychotic for prominent irritability

---

What's the Difference between First- and Second-Generation Antipsychotics?

Essentially, the SGAs developed in the 1990s have fewer and less burdensome side effects than the first-generation antipsychotics (FGAs) like Haldol and Thorazine (chlorpromazine). The FGAs, especially if given long term, can potentially cause wringing of the hands and pursing of the lips as well as stiffness, and they are also more sedating. SGAs act quickly, are less sedating, and generally leave patients more alert. Side effects of SGAs include weight gain, which may be particularly undesirable to teenagers but may be more manageable in younger children. Overall the side effect profile of the two classes of medications makes the SGAs preferable to the FGAs.

Medications do not vary a great deal by bipolar disorder subtype; however, we end up using a medication that addresses depression in type II bipolar disorder, while an SGA often is the first choice for bipolar disorder NOS.

Combination Therapies for Mania

The use of a single mood stabilizer in the treatment of bipolar disorder has been shown to be ineffective in more than 50% of cases. Therefore, your doctor may choose to augment the medication regime with a second mood stabilizer or with an SGA.

Possible medication combinations for mania include:

- Lithium plus one of the antipsychotics (Risperdal, Seroquel, Abilify, Invega, Geodon, Zyprexa, in that order; Abilify precedes other drugs if the child is psychotic)
- Depakote plus one of the antipsychotics
- Trileptal plus one of the antipsychotics (especially if the child is aggressive)
- Lamictal plus one of the antipsychotics (with predominant depressive symptoms)

In cases of severe mania, mania with psychotic features, or treatment resistance, your doctor may start right off combining an antipsychotic with a mood stabilizer such as lithium, Depakote, or Trileptal, then add another mood stabilizer or antipsychotic as needed until the desired results are achieved. This strategy has the advantage of requiring lower doses of SGAs compared to a single-drug therapy, resulting in far fewer severe adverse events. A combination of mood stabilizers, for example, lithium and Depakote, was found to be equally effective in the acute phase, as well as in those who relapsed when put on either of these drugs alone. Excluding those medications that failed to be effective, the doctor can choose the next best option in the list either as an alternative or for a combination regime.

I continue to recommend Trileptal over Tegretol, as it is clinically very effective despite equivocal scientific results. The problem with medication trials in child psychiatry is the lack of a control group that receives placebo treatment for comparison. What parent would agree to have her child participate in a study where she might end up taking a placebo instead of a real active drug for several weeks while she is punching holes in the wall? There are certainly some gracious parents who are committed to research and under thorough medical care do agree, but I must say they are uncommon in my experience.

Guidelines for what to try when faced with chronic resistant symptoms in your child:

1. A single alternative drug.
2. At least two trials of combination regimes of mood stabilizers plus an SGA.
3. Triple therapy addressing comorbid conditions (for example, of additional stimulant for comorbid ADHD). There are no studies in children and adolescents that specifically address the treatment of hypomania, although many children involved in other studies were diagnosed with hypomania. As a rule, treatment of hypomanic symptoms is similar to that of full-blown mania.

Therapy for Depression (Including Treatment Resistance)

A combination of mood stabilizers or SGAs with SSRIs or bupropion has been found to be effective in treating depressed bipolar children. Open studies of lithium, Lamictal, and SGAs alone or in combination in small samples of depressed bipolar youth suggest that this approach may be effective, but randomized clinical trials are needed to confirm these findings.

One study suggested that SSRIs may be helpful for the treatment of depression in teens, but, as mentioned above, SSRIs or other antidepressants may trigger mania, hypomania, mixed episodes, or rapid cycling, particularly when used without concomitant mood stabilizer treatment. The FDA has also required a "black box warning" (a warning printed on the package insert within a bold black border) on antidepressants cautioning parents and professionals to watch for an increase in suicidal thoughts and behaviors among children and teens taking these drugs, particularly early in treatment. This warning followed a review of numerous studies of the drugs that showed an increase in suicidality—*but not actual suicide*—in children with depression and other disorders. It's important to keep in mind that depression itself is associated with an increase in suicidal thoughts and behaviors, so the potential cost–benefit ratio for these medications should be weighed carefully by you and your child's doctor. See page 182 for a discussion of the difficult reality that children with bipolar disorder are at increased risk for suicidality.

For all of the preceding reasons, SSRIs or other antidepressants should be prescribed with caution and in small doses, after stabilization of manic or hypomanic symptoms with mood stabilizers or atypical antipsychotic agents. For example, Lexapro in lower doses such as 2.5 to 5 mg in a time-limited manner and under close supervision and psychoeducation often is effective alongside a mood stabilizer. It is important to balance the risks versus the benefits, given the black box warning associated with SSRI and antidepressant use in children. *One of the most important aspects of treatment for depression among bipolar children is psychosocial therapy (see Chapter 6).*

Therapies for Aggression

We commonly switch patients to an SGA alone if mild aggression is present. In moderate to severe cases, a combination of a mood stabilizer and an SGA is used, working down the list of possible choices after excluding ineffective medications and adequate trials of chosen medications. Catapres (clonidine) can be used to subdue rage attacks when things are out of control, but children can lose their inhibitions or become more aroused after persistent use, although this particular observation needs to be examined further. Sometimes a long-acting drug similar to Catapres, such as Tenex (guanfacine), can work like water on a flame.

The Trials and Tribulations of Medication Management

It can be a long and complicated process to establish a stable medication regimen for a bipolar child. Although it can vary greatly depending on the child's diagnosis, it generally takes about 4 months—and a great deal of patient trial and error—to achieve a basic level of mood stability. And it can take months longer to make the kinds of adjustments needed to maximize functioning and quality of life. To achieve this goal, the physician must have a diverse bag of tricks and good feedback from parents and teachers. Parents need to be able to trust the doctor and commit to trying different strategies, even though some may not work as planned. Here are two examples that illustrate the different paths that may be taken to reach this positive end:

Example 1: Medicating for Multiple Diagnoses and Comorbid Conditions

Eleven-year-old Jack was diagnosed with bipolar disorder, along with a variety of conditions that complicated his treatment, including neuro-cognitive deficits, ADHD, Asperger syndrome, and learning problems. His parents brought him to the clinic after he was put on the antidepressant Lexapro, which made him psychotic—talking to himself and submerged in fantasy—as well as restless and irritable. He also had a history of becoming manic on Concerta, Ritalin, and Adderall. He was overweight already, and his parents did not want him to start on Risperdal given the potential weight gain and prolactin increase.

The first step was to stop Lexapro and start Jack on Seroquel with an aim of increasing the dosage over time. He became increasingly sedated and could not tolerate the medication beyond the initial dose, plus he continued to be psychotic. He was then started on Abilify, which was gradually increased; however, the Abilify caused akathisia (restlessness and an "antsy" feeling), so we needed to add Cogentin to treat this side effect. With the goal of achieving long-term mood stabilization, we also started Jack on a low dose of lithium, which we planned to increase over time.

At this point, Jack was 4 months into his treatment, and, although he stopped hearing voices, he continued to experience rapid mood cycling. His lithium dosage was increased, but, as a result, he felt lethargic and unable to get up in the morning. Therefore, the lithium was split into two doses. Although there was some improvement, he continued to experience mild akathisia despite taking Cogentin. Therefore, his Abilify dosage was decreased as well. Although his rapid mood cycling and psychosis disappeared, he continued to be slow in body and mind, with teachers reporting poor concentration and lethargy at school. Thus, we further reduced both his lithium and Abilify dosages. However, concentrating continued to be a problem. As lithium was on board, we thought it was safe to start Jack on a very small dose of the stimulant Focalin XR (dexmethylphenidate). We increased the stimulant dose to help him concentrate better in school but ended up reducing it after it kept him up at night.

After 8 months of medication management, Jack has blossomed into a confident youngster with a delightful sense of humor and dry wit, able to talk calmly about his realistic concerns in the coming school year, far from the child who came into the clinic months ago.

Example 2: Rebooting the System: Rectifying Medication Overload

Fourteen-year-old Loretta was being managed on multiple medications, including Adderall, Seroquel, Trileptal, Catapres, and Lexapro, plus Inderal (propranolol) at night. She was hospitalized after dancing around naked in response to a high dosage of Adderall. This was an example of what can happen when medications are prescribed one on top of the other without removing previous "misfired" medication regimens from the system. To transition Loretta to a more thoughtful regimen of medication, we rapidly tapered her off all of them over a 1-week period. We would have done this slowly, but given the toxic and serious side effects that could result from such a combination, we chose to do it rapidly on an outpatient basis, keeping close contact with the family.

After she was off the other medications, Loretta was started on lithium slow-release tablets, gradually increasing the dose. Because we didn't expect an immediate improvement, we added a small dose of Risperdal twice a day. As a result, she started to eat enormous amounts of food and gain excessive amounts of weight, so we tapered her off Risperdal. She also continued to feel depressed and was started on Geodon.

After increasing her dosage, she developed extrapyramidal side effects, despite the use of Cogentin on a regular basis. Therefore, Abilify was added, increasing the dosage slowly along with lithium. A stimulant was restarted (much less than the previous dosage and only in the morning), then increased in response to her parents' observation that she appeared to function better on a higher dose. Loretta continued to remain depressed, so Geodon was replaced with Lamictal; and, as she continued to be somewhat lethargic, lithium was gradually stopped.

After 4 months, Loretta has stabilized on a combination of Lamictal, Abilify, and Concerta, which has produced a wonderful balanced mood state without mood cycling, psychosis, or depressive symptoms. And we were able to avoid antidepressants, which was especially important given her negative response to these medications in the past.

Alternative and Complementary Treatments

Because available medications don't do everything for every child, there's a strong call for additional new interventions. If you, like many parents, find natural alternatives highly appealing and acceptable, you'll be interested to know that the most promising alternative treatments for bipolar disorder in children are the omega-3 fatty acids.

Omega-3 Fatty Acids

The evidence in favor of omega-3 fatty acids is encouraging but preliminary and suggests the need for well-designed, adequately powered, randomized controlled trials. However, medical consensus is developing that prescribing them is justified for depressive patients not responding optimally to standard treatment for mood instability. Side effects are mild and rare and can include fishy aftertaste, gastrointestinal disturbance, altered bleeding time, and lowered glucose levels.

Omega-3 fatty acids play an important role in normal brain development and function and have potential relevance to a wide range of psychiatric, developmental, and neurological disorders. The typical American diet is too low in omega-3 fats compared to omega-6 fats, and this relative disappearance of omega-3 fats from the diet in developed countries has been linked with increases in a wide range of both physical and mental disorders. Fortunately, omega-3 fatty acids are available in fish and fish oil and also seeds, green vegetables, and nuts. Currently, the American Heart Association recommends that those without heart disease should eat at least two servings of fatty fish per week along with other foods rich in omega-3 fatty acids, which appears to be safe for everyone in this broad population.

Studies of omega-3 fatty acids as an add-on therapy have shown that they not only alleviate bipolar symptoms but also help prevent mood swings, decrease irritability, and increase the time between bipolar episodes. They also seem to have a positive effect on depression in both adults and children. Omega-3 fatty acids confer an additive advantage of improving the attention deficits and impulsivity that so many bipolar children experience as well, without precipitating or worsening manic symptoms as other treatments for ADHD can—for instance, with S-adenosyl methionine (SAM-e), another popular supplement used to manage depressive symptoms in those with bipolar disorder and ADHD. Most treatment trials of fatty acids have used doses of around 400–1,600 mg of the fatty acids known as EPA and DHA in varying ratios for bipolar disorder and 300–700 mg of these two for ADHD. Ask your child's doctor whether omega-3 supplements could be helpful in your child's case.

Lecithin (Phosphatidylcholine) and Choline

Bipolar teenagers have been found to have lowered choline levels in the medial orbitofrontal cortex region of the brain, and the active form of lecithin, phosphatidylcholine, is a major component of cell membranes. Several studies have shown lecithin/choline to reduce mania (including in one teenager who took lecithin/phosphatidylcholine for more than 2 years without symptoms after stopping lithium), though additional controlled studies are needed to confirm these effects. Side effects seem to be minor and to be mainly nausea, vomiting, and diarrhea. But, if your child's doctor agrees to augment medication treatment with lecithin or choline, the dose should start low and be increased only gradually. (Also note that these supplements seemed to increase depression in those with unipolar, not bipolar, depression.)

S-Adenosyl Methionine (SAM-e)

A few controlled preliminary studies have shown that this supplement, available on the market in the United States since 1999 and for much longer in Europe, may help alleviate depression in bipolar disorder. However, at higher doses SAM-e may exacerbate mania and depression in those with bipolar disorder, and it has drug interactions that are of concern. Besides gastrointestinal side effects, it may cause insomnia, nervousness, headache, dizziness, dry mouth, sweating, or heart palpitations. So it should be considered only under the very careful supervision of a child's prescribing physician and generally only for treatment-resistant depression, at least until further research has been done.

Inositol

Inositol, informally referred to as vitamin B_8, may ease symptoms of depression when taken along with lithium. Gastrointestinal side effects like nausea and diarrhea have been reported, and there are drug interactions to be aware of with high doses of this supplement.

Others

L-tryptophan has been shown in some studies—though almost all on adults—to reduce mania in bipolar individuals, especially as a supplement to lithium, but this supplement may cause a variety of side effects and drug interactions, and whether the evidence in favor of L-tryptophan can be extended to adolescents and children is questionable. Taurine may have potential for reducing mania, particularly in those with rapid-cycling bipolar disorder, but research is still preliminary. Vitamins have often been claimed to be important in mood regulation, and research has shown that deficiencies in vitamins such as B_1, B_6, B_{12}, and C may contribute to depression, but megavitamin treatment for children is dubious at best, as I explain below.

Bogus Treatments

As mentioned, there are bogus assessments and there are also bogus treatments. Being married to a pediatrician/neonatologist, I am continually warned that too many vitamins in high doses are harmful for babies and children. Megavitamin therapy, supplying multiple minerals, and detoxification are all inappropriate in my view, no matter what you may have read about these complementary or alternative "treatments." When all is said and done, a subset of bipolar children may have poor immunity, get migraines easily, and be generally fragile. It won't hurt to give these children an over-the-counter vitamin B and C combination.

However, when families talk about alternatives such as pranic healing, a so-called no-touch energy healing in which the body is assisted in healing itself, I worry. There is no evidence that this approach can help anyone with bipolar disorder. Other alternatives, such as homeopathy, may have complementary merit when delivered by someone fully trained, with a degree in homeopathy, but any bogus doctor setting up a specialized clinic to give homeopathic pills can be useless, if not harmful.

Herbs like St. John's wort contain components similar to antidepressants, which, as you now know, can worsen mania. St. John's wort can have the same negative effects if you decide to give it to your child for depression thinking it is a natural product and therefore must be harmless at worst. Natural products do not equate with safe, healthy products!

You've probably heard about light therapy for winter depression (seasonal affective disorder, or SAD), and it works for some people with this type of depression, but it should not be used routinely for bipolar children. It is an uncommon strategy to use but not actually bogus.

Some of my favorite moms and dads swear by the miracles worked by alternative medicines. When I do not know of any trials that would support their use, I say so, but parents often end up making their own choice after listening to me. I like to advise parents but give them space.

Treating Comorbid Conditions

"Even when [my child's] mood is stable, symptoms of comorbid disorders such as ADHD and ODD interfere with her functioning. What keeps me hopeful: Her moods are mostly stable with the combo of meds she is now on."

Very often, a "rescue" medication is needed in addition to the primary mood stabilizer to treat symptoms such as aggression, psychosis, and sleep disturbance. This same situation can apply to ADHD, anxiety, or other comorbid conditions.

Comorbid ADHD

While ADHD is a distinct disorder separate from childhood bipolar disorder, it is not understood whether the ADHD-like symptoms in bipolar disorder warrant additional treatment beyond mood stabilization. In our research studies and clinic, several patients continued to show symptoms of inattention after mood stabilization that warranted the addition of stimulant medication. Cognitive difficulties such as shifting attention and executive function seen in both ADHD and bipolar disorder can potentially be addressed by stimulants. Stimulants are almost always given in long-acting form unless an additional after-school dose is required to sustain the benefits.

Among psychostimulants, long-acting methylphenidate (such as Ritalin compounds) or mixed amphetamine salts are equally effective. Strattera is an alternative treatment if stimulants have been ineffective, although there are no data establishing the safety or efficacy of Strattera in treating bipolar children with comorbid ADHD. Strattera is a selective norepinephrine reuptake inhibitor with potential antidepressant effects that could theoretically trigger or exacerbate manic symptoms, so it should be used with great care in bipolar children.

Comorbid Anxiety

Anxiety disorders, including generalized anxiety disorder and separation anxiety disorder, are relatively common, especially in bipolar type I. Psychotherapeutic interventions such as CBT remain the first choice of treatment in children and adolescents with comorbid bipolar disorder and anxiety disorder. Small doses of SSRIs such as Lexapro as adjuvant medication may be effective if mania is stabilized, though there are no controlled trials for anxiety comorbid with bipolar disorder. SSRIs are the only medications consistently shown to be effective in controlled trials for childhood anxiety disorders. This treatment intervention requires educating the family about the risk of a manic switch, and close monitoring of the treatment response is necessary. Tenex may also be a choice if vigilance, arousal, and excitability are prominent. Benzodiazepines and BuSpar (buspirone) follow as alternative choices. The risk for developing dependence needs to be considered for long-term use of benzodiazepines in adolescents. BuSpar may not be effective in all cases. Inderal may be considered in cases of performance anxiety. Medication is often utilized in small doses to reduce risks of exacerbating bipolar disorder and to enable patients to benefit from psychotherapeutic interventions.

How Do We Deal with Medication Problems?

Side Effects

Low doses and slow titration (building up the medication gradually in the bloodstream) are two fundamental principles that can help minimize adverse reactions to medication. If problems continue, switching to an alternative medication may be necessary. You may decide that the benefit of the offending drug outweighs the negatives. In that case, an effort must be made to continue it at the desired dose with appropriate management strategies. For example, you may have seen excellent response only with lithium, but your son develops low thyroid levels. We can treat this side effect with synthetic thyroid supplement and continue lithium. If your daughter responds only to Risperdal but has tremendous weight gain, we can lower the dose and try nutrition and weight management. Here are some other tips for dealing with common side effects:

Weight Gain

There are lots of ideas promoted for losing weight, but the single most important intervention is diet and exercise. Weight Watchers online, especially when followed along with a parent, is an inexpensive and effective choice. Timely meals and wise food choices reduce excessive calories. Avoid sodas. Cut down on junk food. Provide healthy snacks. If weight gain continues to be a problem, avoid Zyprexa and preferably use Geodon or Lamictal as alternatives. Adding Topamax as an adjuvant in low doses sometimes works, but tingling and numbing of peripheral nerves is a possible complication, although not very common.

Involuntary Movements

These are a common side effect of antipsychotic medications, mostly from FGAs, but can occur with SGAs too, as previously discussed in this chapter. Symptoms can include involuntary movements, tremors and rigidity, body restlessness (akathisia), muscle contractions, and changes in breathing and heart rate. Cogentin 1–2 mg every other day to once a day is effective in combating these symptoms. Akathisia in patients treated with SGAs is often overlooked and may respond to low doses of Inderal.

Sedation

While they help moderate mood, some medications can also make your child drowsy. Nighttime dosing decreases problems with sedation, and it is customary for the clinician to take advantage of that fact by increasing the dose of a sedating mood stabilizer at bedtime. Beyond that, melatonin 1–3 mg, Gabitril (tiagabine) 2–4 mg, or trazodone 25–50 mg can be administered to establish the sleep routine that is critical for bipolar children. While these compounds have not been specifically tested on bipolar youth, they are known to work, be safe in the pediatric population, and interfere minimally with REM sleep. In subjects with abuse potential, benzodiazepines may be misused and medications such as Trazodone may be effective alternatives.

Gastrointestinal Symptoms

Long-acting preparations of Depakote or lithium, or taking SGA at night before bed, tend to decrease gastrointestinal upset.

Lithium-Related High Thyroid Stimulating Hormone (TSH)

An endocrine consultation is needed to evaluate for hypothyroidism, which may or may not be related to lithium use. If lithium needs to be continued, hypothyroidism can be effectively treated with levothyroxine 25–50 mcg a day, titrated based on levels of TSH on follow-up.

Rash

A rash is usually associated with Trileptal or Lamictal. Starting these drugs at low doses and titrating up the dose at very low increments can help avoid rash, especially with Lamictal. Lamictal is titrated up at 12.5 mg a week over 6–12 weeks to get to desirable level (150–400 mg).

Bedwetting (Enuresis)

If this is associated with taking Risperdal, usually adding an anticholinergic agent leads to improvement. If the problem is caused by lithium and specific gravity of early morning urine is not low, desmopressin (DDAVP) is safe to use. Overall, DDAVP, if taken up to two puffs in each nostril before bedtime, can save loads of blankets being washed each day. More important, DDAVP can be useful at sleepovers.

Despite the many benefits that medication offers the bipolar child, there's a lot we don't know. More research is needed to take the guesswork out of treating childhood bipolar disorder—I mean clinical research, rather than animal studies that translate to human physiology. We need real proof of what is effective for children in real-life practice!

Managing Medications in Real Life

In addition to dealing with the physical effects, parents are challenged by the daily logistical and psychological aspects of medication management. For instance, what do you do if your child won't (or can't) take his or her medication? How do you handle medication on overnight visits, at school, or on trips? What happens if your child has an adverse reaction to a medication when you're not there? Here are a few suggestions to help you maintain your medication program and deal with the unforeseen issues that may come up:

- *If you forget a medication,* it is best to move on to the next dosing and not try to correct it by taking a double dose the next time around, as a general rule. If your child is off medication for several weeks, starting the drug at full dose abruptly may be too hard to cope with. That can be dangerous, especially in the case of Lamictal, where a restarted heavy dose after a gap without a slow increase can cause a rash.
- *If your child cannot swallow pills,* there are patches or meltaway tablets for use under the tongue, elixirs, or spansules you can pour out as sprinkles on applesauce to make medication easier to take. These preparations for each medication are summarized in the *Handbook of Psychopharmacotherapy* listed in Resources.

- *When your child is away from home overnight*, such as at a sleepover, he can protect his privacy once he's old enough to handle his own medications (generally at around age 12), carrying them in a zippered bag in his pocket and taking the pills privately. If he's staying at the home of a trusted relative like a favorite aunt or his best friend's mom, the medications can be entrusted to that adult, which is a good alternative for kids under age 12. Note that summer camps require nurses to administer such medications.

Paying for Medication

"If I have blood work done to check my child's lithium level, the medical insurance folks won't pay for it because it is for mental health, and the mental health insurance folks reject the claim, saying it is a medical expense. I went through a year of getting claims rejected by both and bounced back and forth; ultimately, I had to pay it all myself."

Children with bipolar disorder can take multiple drugs and may require close monitoring that involves numerous tests and doctors' visits. Paying for this can present a challenge, especially as many insurance plans will pay for some, but not all, of the medications, testing, and follow-up that are needed. If you have limited or no insurance, here are a few ideas for how you can get help paying for your child's medications and related treatment costs.

Get into a Study

If you are fortunate to live near an academic medical center, or are willing to travel to one, your child may be eligible to participate in a treatment study geared to children with bipolar disorder. Essentially, you get free excellent diagnostic assessment and careful monitoring of treatment for a time-limited period. Most of these types of programs take responsibility to connect you with the best available follow-up clinical care soon after the trial.

Fortunately, more funding has been allocated for research in pediatric bipolar disorder in the past few years, and this has made clinical research possible in this previously neglected area. Research studies typically investigate a new medication or therapy and compare it to old treatments or other types of treatment. When you and your child consent to participate in the study, any therapy or medication used is typically free for the duration of the study. While in the study, your child is typically seen frequently and monitored, but some elements of his care may not be addressed. Some families have used study participation for second opinions, for treatment, or as a bridge to extend insurance coverage when it has been appropriate and acceptable for their child's treatment and of interest to the child. CABF has a list of studies open to children on its website (*www.bpkids.org*), and often travel expenses are covered. You can also check with NIMH (*www.nimh.nih.gov*), or by searching through Google. Not all studies are listed on websites as it costs money to advertise them. Your best bet may be to call the regional university hospital or mental health system near you that is a known research center for bipolar disorder, such as the Pediatric Mood Disorders Clinic at the University of Illinois at Chicago (*www.psych.uic.edu*) that I direct, to ask if there are any ongoing research studies that may suit your child.

Does Your State Require Mental Health Parity?

Ask your insurance company whether your child's diagnosis of bipolar disorder requires the company to provide mental health benefits equivalent (same copays, deductibles, etc.) to those for a medical condition. This concept is known as *parity* and is mandated to a degree by federal law and by state law in about two thirds of states as of 2007, and there is new legislation pending designed to expand these options. Exactly how similar mental health benefits must be varies from state to state. The American Academy of Child and Adolescent Psychiatry keeps close track of developments in such areas; its website (*aacap.org*) is a good place to consult for more detailed, up-to-date information.

Ask for Medication Samples

Doctors typically can offer medication samples to families starting new medications or those with a child who is taking so many different medications that the out-of-pocket costs are astronomical. Because of the complex nature of bipolar disorder and common co-occurring disorders like ADHD, families may have three, four, five, or more different medications with separate copays for each. My coworkers and I have been told by many working insured families that their medication copays can sometimes exceed hundreds of dollars a month. We are sensitive to this plight and try to problem-solve with our drug representatives and with drug companies about solutions for these types of problems, and we know how expensive medications can be if you do not have insurance! Our experience is that drug reps and drug companies want to help and have at times provided us with vouchers for a month of free trial medications or with more samples because of these situations. However, most doctors have limited access to samples, so you may need to educate them about your medication expenses and needs so that they can help you find ways of keeping effective medications accessible. There are also ways of spreading out your prescriptions. For instance, some pills can be split so that, if your doctor orders a larger dose, one pill can actually be two doses, making a single prescription last twice as long. This is not always possible, but brainstorm with your doctor for ideas on economical ways to get the medications your child needs.

Explore No-Cost or Low-Cost Medication Options

Each pharmaceutical company has a low- or no-cost medications program for families in need. Your doctor, your doctor's drug reps, and pharmaceutical companies' websites can help you get updated information on these programs and locate applications. Each company has its own rules and policies. Some send medications directly to your doctor; others may send them directly to you if you meet program criteria. The Pharmaceutical Research and Manufacturers of America publication order line is another good resource (see the facing page), and pharmaceutical companies sometimes list low- or no-cost medication programs on their websites. Again, follow through and be persistent with any of these strategies, and let your doctor know what you are doing so that he or she can help.

Another way to keep medication costs low is to see if generic forms are available for the medications your child takes. Generic forms of medications can be 20–40% lower in cost than brand names, if they are available. It doesn't hurt to ask. Newer medications are less likely to have generic forms, as it takes a while for them to be developed and get approval from the necessary regulatory agencies. Let your doctor know if you prefer generics or brand names.

Families can also save money on prescriptions by using a mail-order pharmacy service. This requires your doctor to write a prescription for a 90-day supply of drugs rather than a monthly prescription and that the refill be for a 3-month period. This can be helpful in reducing copays (as you eliminate two of them by having 90 days' worth dispensed at once rather than several times over 3 months) but may not be an option if you are still trying to get the right medication combination or tweaking dosages.

No- or Low-Cost Medication Programs

Call the Pharmaceutical Research and Manufacturers of America publication order line (1-202-835-3450) to request their Patient Assistance Directory, or go online to *www.pharma.org*

Beyond Medication: The Role of Therapy in Childhood Bipolar Disorder

Although we'd all love a magic pill, medication alone cannot address all the bipolar child's needs. While medication will help stabilize mood swings, other interventions are needed to monitor your child's mood and help her cope with the day-to-day environment. Other interventions can ensure that your child gets the maximum benefit possible from the medications. As everyone around the child is affected by the disorder, treatment must include the whole family. Chapter 6 talks about how to maintain your child's mood and help him and the rest of the family function better with therapy and behavior management.

SIX

Making Life Better
with RAINBOW Therapy

"Hope for us comes in a lot of forms. Some days it is as small as a smile on a day that has otherwise been generally hard. This can be like finding the pot of gold at the end of a rainbow. . . . Two members of my family are blessed with the insights that bipolar disorder can often bring. I feel that having their input and knowing when they struggle and how they triumph helps us all survive better."

"Without our intervention (therapy, medicines, counseling), she would not have [this] quality of life. . . . I remain hopeful that one day she'll manage this herself and she'll be able to mentor others and contribute to society in a positive and compassionate way."

Why Is Therapy Important, and What Kind Do We Need?

Few scientists or doctors would argue with the importance of medication in the management of childhood bipolar disorder. In fact, medication management has become the current standard of care for both children and adults. However, because of the complexity of the disorder and your child's changing psychology and physiology as he grows, there is always a risk of relapse, even with careful medication management. The need for other therapy goes beyond the goal of maximizing the positive effects of medication; as this chapter will show, you're going to need both therapy and medication to cope and thrive on a daily basis.

In my treatment and research, I've observed that other methods of intervention are necessary to prolong and sustain treatment improvements. My own studies indicate that a particular form of "psychosocial interventions" that combines medication with education about the nature of bipolar disorder—child- and family-focused cognitive-behavioral therapy (CBT) —benefits bipolar children in a number of ways. If you think of it in terms of building a house, then medication management is like the foundation, psychological counseling the bricks, and family therapy the cement that helps hold it all together. This kind of therapy helps a bipolar child develop a positive self-concept, learn better coping methods, and establish healthy social relationships, improving quality of life and preventing relapse.

Because it's easy for children and families to remember, as I mentioned in the introduction, I call this treatment method RAINBOW, symbolizing the happiness and calm that often comes after the storm and serving as a beacon of hope to families in turmoil due to bipolar disorder. RAINBOW is also in keeping with my philosophy that mood variability (represented by the colors of the rainbow) is appropriate in moderation (green versus "ultraviolet" sad moods or "infrared" rages or manic spells, which are more extreme). In my practice, I work with families on incorporating the RAINBOW system into their daily lives, with the aim of helping the bipolar child reach the safe middle zone I describe below. See the box for an overview of RAINBOW.

Study Results: RAINBOW Offers Hope

Using a systematic protocol, we initially evaluated the effectiveness of RAINBOW therapy on 36 children in our clinic through a research protocol. After treatment, there were improvements in symptoms of mania, depression, psychosis, aggression, inattention, and sleep difficulties. Overall functioning improved and rapid cycling decreased from 97.1% before treatment to 32.4% after receiving it. While we await future systematic trials, this one gave us hope that this approach makes a difference in the lives of bipolar children and their families. Subsequently, we went on to use this method with incredible success in hundreds of children. We also followed the children over 3 years and found that the effects of this treatment were sustained with families receiving booster follow-up treatment. The incidence of mania, depression, aggression, psychosis, sleep disturbances, and ADHD decreased, and overall functioning improved.

Key Ingredients of RAINBOW Therapy:
For You and Your Child

- *R* **for Routine:** Establish a strict routine to encourage a stable schedule while cutting down on negotiation that can produce conflict and distraction.
- *A* **for Affect (mood) regulation/Anger control:** Teach the child to use mood charts to monitor his or her emotional state. Parents and other family members should understand the cyclical nature of the disorder and the role of medications in controlling large and frequent mood swings seen in bipolar children.
- *I* **for "I can do it":** Encourage the child to tell a positive self-story and make positive self-statements at home and school to encourage and build self-esteem. You, too, ought to learn to give yourself positive feedback.
- *N* **for "No negative thoughts":** Restructure negative thinking by guiding the child to think of how to change unhelpful thoughts or experiences at school to helpful ones that would make a difference. You should also focus on positive, constructive thoughts. "Live in the *now*" is the mantra for coping by living in the moment, otherwise referred to as mindfulness.
- *B* **for Be a good friend/Balanced lifestyle:** Proactively teach your child to make friendships and, more important, keep those friendships. This will foster a sense of self-worth and connectedness to peers. "Belonging" is important to feeling good. Given the demands of "being on" all the time to help your child, it is important to seek a balanced lifestyle for yourself, too.
- *O* **for Optimal problem solving:** Family members are encouraged to engage in collaborative problem solving with children, but they should wait until rages pass. *Important note: Immediate consequences for undesirable behavior are* **not** *recommended, and reward systems should be used with moderation. Teaching through "pep talks" is the key to influencing bipolar children.*
- *W* **for "Ways to get support":** Children are encouraged to draw a support tree and put the names of all the people whom they could reach out to and are close to them on each branch. This technique is intended to help children recognize that they have a supportive safety network or system around them to nurture them when they are in need.

RAINBOW therapy, which we deliver at our clinic in 12 sessions, also helps address other issues that commonly interfere with recovery, such as anxiety, ADHD, and developmental problems including poor regulation and impulse control. Thus, children learn the importance of taking medications and are more apt to remain in treatment. The last but most important reason to participate in RAINBOW treatment is that you get to learn the tips to continue the therapeutic environment at home and foster your child's growth as she matures. You are not in the dark, leaving while your therapist spends an hour a week with your child and doesn't tell you what is going on. You become involved, skilled, and in control. Knowing you can do something, knowing you did all you could, and knowing the limitations of how much you can do is so liberating! This kind of therapy is not just for your child, but also for you.

Although RAINBOW therapy is my own creation with my team, the principles behind it can be used with any form of therapy. Even if you can't find the same program in your community, you can share this philosophy and these tools with your doctors and use these principles to help manage bipolar disorder at home.

How Does RAINBOW Therapy Work?

There are several practices associated with CFF-CBT that form the backbone of RAINBOW treatment for childhood bipolar disorder. These practices are designed to help the child with bipolar disorder establish routine, monitor and manage mood swings, improve self-esteem and coping ability, reduce negative thinking and anxiety, build social skills, engage in effective problem solving, and seek social support when appropriate. The following pages give you an idea of what we do in our clinic, along with lots of practical suggestions for adopting the principles and strategies at home. While these strategies must be reinforced and applied with the help of a therapist to be fully effective, they can be implemented as self-help too.

Establishing Routine

I don't have to tell you that life is chaos with a bipolar child in the family. You already know that, if you let them, bipolar children will get up late, watch TV all day, and eat and socialize or not socialize as they please! But what I want to remind you is that establishing a normal life to the greatest extent possible, setting up pillars of strength and anchors of guidance, will help you kick-start manageable days. By routine I mean much more than regular meal and bedtimes, though those practical routines are certainly important. I highly encourage all families to aim for what one mother called "consistency with each other," meaning paying attention to treating each other with respect and in the same way from day to day. Then your child can count on a level of emotional stability around him.

The All-Important Sleep Cycle

That said, the overarching goal of routine is to get the sleep cycle into a healthy pattern, as I've said before. If that cycle is disturbed, it can trigger a fluctuating mood state interspersed with rages. So, it is preventive and stabilizing to have a good night's sleep every single day. This will reduce tiredness and abnormal shifts in circadian rhythm and help make transitions between activities much smoother.

Bipolar children will often push the limits with bedtime—particularly if they are in a manic or hypomanic phase, especially as decreased need for sleep is a common symptom of illness. The therapist should be able to help you find behavioral strategies to establish or reestablish the sleep routine so your child is rested and able to function during the day. Some of these may include taking a shower or drinking milk that may cue her to the upcoming ritual of receiving your bedtime kiss and/or a back rub. Avoid mental stimulation or activities like computer games or caffeine-based drinks such as sodas or coffee. Consistency in bedtime, wake-up time, and bedtime routines is extremely important. Turn the TV off, keep noise levels down, and switch off the lights. Do not let weekends throw you off. Keep the routine the same (well, almost) during holidays and weekends. A good rule is to set bedtimes no more than 1 hour later on weekends and 2 hours later during summer vacations, making it easier to reestablish the school-day routine.

I know of a child who slept as soon as he came home from school. His mother thought he was tired and let him sleep. This is often the case because some medications sedate children and they tire trying to stay tuned in at school. Try to minimize naps by adjusting the medications as well as limiting naptime to no more than 30 minutes to an hour, but only if it is a must. I am not suggesting naps as necessary or allowed if they aren't needed. I also think it is OK to change medications if poor sleep is becoming a persistent problem. There are several options that you can ask your doctor for, and some are mentioned in the section of Chapter 5 on prescribing the right medications.

Regular Meals and Snacks

Another element of the routine to pay attention to is diet. Did you ever hear the saying "A hungry man is an angry man"? Hunger, autonomic instability (that underlies the excitability and agitation), and sleep disturbance are all linked in the brain through a brain structure called the hypothalamus. So feed your child regularly and on time.

Relaxing Activities

Apart from maintaining a daily schedule, also think of factoring in a couple of activities during the week to soothe your child. For example, swimming and tennis are good choices that are not contact sports and can be manageable either alone or with a partner. They serve as "release" activities. Soft music will *help your child release tension and soothe himself*. Lots of mothers have told us this is a great way to help their kids relax that is readily accepted any day. Ultimately, it is highly individual as to what calms a child. See Chapter 8 for more ways to set up flexible routines that can help the family function better at home.

Consistent but Not Rigid

Don't make your routines too rigid or you'll find yourself going crazy trying to keep everyone on task. Don't increase your stress by trying too hard! Pick important times in the day that include wake-up time, school time, dinnertime, homework time, and bedtime and stick to them religiously. You being there around the time your child wakes up may be the single most important thing to start him or her off nicely. And be kind to yourself (see Chapter 7 for tips).

Affect Regulation: Managing Moods

I find it can be helpful to look upon your child's moods as a rainbow, ranging from "ultraviolet" sad moods on one end to "infrared" rages or manic spells on the other. The goal is to help your child spend as much time as possible in the safe green zones in the middle of the spectrum. Your child will be the hardest to help when her moods are at the outer edges of this spectrum. Often, I ask families and children to describe their experience with mood fluctuations. One teen described her mood disorder as like an "invisible fist" that hits her. Naming the experience of the disorder will help your child remember that it's something separate from her; bipolar disorder doesn't define her.

As I explained in Chapter 5, one goal of medication is stabilizing your child's moods to stay in the center range (between 1 and 4 out of an extreme of 10 in either a high or low direction; see the figure below). Medication is like a plaster to a broken arm. Bones won't set unless you leave the plaster on. Similarly, if your child won't take medication, bones can get infected and heal in the wrong position or not at all. In the same way, other mental problems can accrue if we don't take care of bipolar disorder *now*. So, stressing the need to take medication, even when your child doesn't want to, is a key step toward mood regulation.

What Parents Can Say to Overcome Medication Resistance

One of the best ways to help overcome medication resistance is through diplomacy—treat your child like a partner, use logic, and bring the doctor into it to help problem-solve. Here are some examples of how you can accomplish this feat:

- *"I know it's a chore to take it each day, but think of it like a vitamin pill that you need to take, and JUST DO IT!"*
- *"The more we fuss about it, the harder it gets, honey. I will stand*

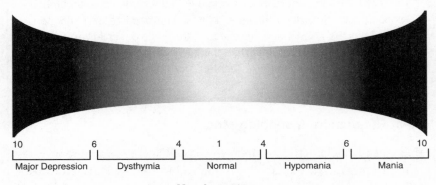

10	6	4	1	4	6	10
Major Depression	Dysthymia		Normal		Hypomania	Mania

Mood spectrum.

right by you each day and help you until it becomes no big deal. How about that?"

- *"I know you hate medication, but it is a necessary evil that helps you enjoy life a lot more."*
- *"I know that you don't like feeling sleepy with the pills. How about I speak to the doctor and we will adjust it so you don't feel so tired, OK?"*
- *"I know you suffer way more than me or anyone in our family. As much as you don't want to deal with pills, they help you relax and feel better. If they are not working, we will talk to the doctor and adjust them so they really help you, darling."*
- *"I know pills are large or you hate pills or you don't like taking so many. How about we talk and discuss it with the doctor to learn how we can make it the best possible regime or type of pills?"*

In an emergency, you may need to administer an "as needed" medication to prevent an escalating mood swing. Under these circumstances, it is better to say kindly, "How about a relaxing pill for you, sweetheart?" rather than stiffly interjecting, "I see you getting manic. You have to take the pill to stop that right now."

One goal of CFF-CBT is to teach parents how to communicate effectively with their bipolar child and use influence, rather than confrontation or control. This technique is the best way to curtail disruptive, aggressive, or insolent behavior that can erupt during "red" periods and provide behavioral strategies for balancing compassion with firm boundaries during other times. As I've said earlier, tell yourself, "Be strong," when your child is in that zone. When she calls you names, remember it's the disorder talking and administer firm but gentle correction.

Using Mood Charts

"Keep a journal of your child's behaviors, moods, treatments, appointments, reactions, triggers, etc.," advises one parent. "This information is invaluable as you move forward. Even today, 6 years after diagnosis of my first child with bipolar disorder, I find this record immensely helpful." I encourage you to keep mood charts on your child's emotional state for several reasons: first, it helps your child understand himself by looking at the chart. Eventually, this tool works as a feedback mechanism to recognize and preempt pending mood swings. Second, mood charts provide a visual analogue when starting a new medication, as they help you see and monitor the results. Finally, they help educate your child and other members of your family about the cyclical nature of the disorder. It can help siblings realize, "Oh, that's what's going on with my sister," rather than teasing or lashing out, although sometimes siblings can start to point out or exaggerate the troubles, creating problems rather than helping prevent them. So be on the lookout for negative input from siblings, and use the charts wisely based on your situation. Mood charts can also be useful at school to help teachers and other school personnel better understand your child's condition and determine the best ways to address her needs. More about working with school personnel can be found in Chapter 9.

Mood charts can be extremely simple. You can just take a regular calendar and color in the moods on a daily or weekly basis to denote whether that day or week was sad or withdrawn (blue), normal (green), or angry, excitable, or aggressive (red). Over time, your child will learn how to maintain this chart for herself. As she begins to understand her fluctuating moods and identify the warning signs of a mood swing, you both will be in a better position to seek medical assistance early or employ positive self-talk and other techniques to prevent a meltdown. See Appendix G

Mood Monitoring and Management

- Sit down with your child and update the mood chart on a daily or weekly basis, depending on your child's typical cycles.
- Emphasize the positive by embracing your child's unique personality and emotional shadings, making it clear that the goal is to help her be happy and calm, not change who she is.
- Don't wait until the situation becomes extreme to act. Intervene at the first indication that your child is leaving the middle (green) zone. Therapy can help parents employ effective communication techniques and boundary setting under these circumstances.
- Keep your child's doctor, therapist, and other support professionals updated on your child's status by sharing the mood chart with them frequently. This can be especially useful during medication trials.
- Use the chart to help educate family members, close friends, teachers, and coaches about bipolar disorder and how they can be supportive of your child in difficult times.

Don't Make the Mood Chart Your Life's Work

Keep a mood chart only if you feel you and your child are able to do it. I believe that these tasks should help rather than hinder progress or create more work for you. Often, parents bring me bundles of charts and journals neatly put together into a binder with dozens of colors documenting every little mood change. While I understand that it can be cathartic and help give you perspective, for some people this can seem like an overwhelming chore. How much time and detailed attention you want to put into a mood chart depends on what is best for *you*. But keep your eyes on the big picture. Always remember the first point in your new philosophy (see Chapter 4): Take the pressure off!

---

for a sample daily mood calendar. There are also several samples of mood charts available at the CABF website, *www.bpkids.org.*

"I Can Do It": Improving Self-Esteem

Bipolar children often have a poor self-image because of the way people, especially peers, react to their unpredictable and bossy behavior. This is compounded, of course, by the likelihood of learning problems leading to academic failure. Because of their extreme sensitivity to criticism, they often see themselves as helpless victims. This leads to a range of maladaptive behaviors, such as lying or risk taking, to cover up feelings of inadequacy and hopelessness.

There are several important things you can do right now to foster a positive self-image and bolster your child's sense of self. As we discussed earlier, you serve as a mirror to help your child internalize a positive message about himself. Here's a list to get you started:

1. *Equip your child with at least five positive self-statements.* By that, I mean tell him five things you love and admire about him. Get him to pick some statements about himself, too. Keep trying to catch him being good whenever you can! Let your child see himself in a positive light through your eyes.

2. *Give your child gentle pep talks while you teach her.* (Say, "You can do it!" in different ways to help her learn to say, "I can do it!") Get

your boy to have play dates with Dad and your girl to have play dates with Mom. Value your child's company and give her attention while teaching her skills that she can take pride in. Play chess at the local coffee shop as you buy hot chocolate, or take your child for a walk.

3. *For at least for 5 minutes a day, look into your child's eyes and just listen to what he has to say. I call this "5-Minute Magic Tonic."*

4. *Get your child to write positive stories about herself* in which she can describe what is special, great, or amazing about herself, her interests, and her achievements. These stories can become a treasure chest from which your child can draw strength whenever she likes.

5. *Change your child's perception of himself* by helping him find positive outlets and activities, and identify and appreciate his personal islands of competence, a subject, sport, game, or hobby that he does well in and can look upon with pride. Get your child involved in a sport he likes or is potentially good at that he can do by himself, with no contact and a limited number of partners. Swimming, tennis, golf, and even track or dance may be appropriate.

Think in terms of *"projective identification."* Does it sound like psychoanalytic mumbo jumbo? It is, but with a profound meaning. I often tell parents that if we expect positive things from our children, we must also treat them well. If we believe in them, trust them, and enjoy them, they are more likely to respond in kind. Project the image, and they will identify with it and act accordingly! Expect and believe in positive behavior. It may not always work, but keep trying, especially when your child is in a stable mood. A positive outlook and looking for the good in your child will help your mood as well and help create a less stressful atmosphere that allows positive things to happen.

Tips for Building Your Child's Self-Esteem

- Give your child a list of five things you love about him or her.
- Help your child write a list of five things he likes about himself.
- Encourage your child to write positive stories about herself that she can reread when she needs a boost.

- Tell your child, "You can do it!" till he's in the habit of saying, "I can do it!"
- Spend at least 5 minutes a day listening to your child with your undivided attention.
- Promote your child's talents and skills with activities that take advantage of them.
- Teach your child to soothe himself with things he likes—and offer back rubs to soothe him yourself.
- Get your child involved in solo sports to build her sense of competence.
- Help your child believe in herself by showing that you believe in her.

Parents Need a Shot of Self-Esteem, Too!

Remember that these strategies work exactly the same way to help you feel good about yourself. Practice saying positive things to yourself. Give yourself credit for making the effort to learn all there is to learn to help your child by reading this book. Give yourself a pat on the back for trying so hard. You are my star!

No Negative Thoughts: Eliminating Negative Thinking

Continuing struggles with school, friends, and even other family members can produce a pretty negative outlook and a tendency to project negative thoughts and attitudes into the future. It's easy to see why bipolar children are apt to say, "I can never win" and "Nobody will ever like me." By employing the techniques of CBT, the bipolar child can come to recognize that he is not the only one who has struggles, failures, and losses. The bipolar child is not alone! Helping him realize that no one gets everything he wants or is liked by everyone can help normalize these daily struggles. Helping him recognize and nurture the successes and friendships he already has will help shift the focus to the here and now. This can open the door to realistic solutions, such as tutoring in a difficult subject.

Have several ideas ready to help combat negative thoughts. Teach your child to say "stop" to negative thoughts. Reframe hardships to find tangible solutions. Teach her to think of alternatives immediately. Get

---

How to Help Your Child Change Negative Thoughts into Positive Outcomes

1. Teach your child to look at problems as opportunities to practice problem-solving skills.
2. Encourage your child to identify the source of the problem immediately and come up with alternative solutions.
3. Have your child write down solutions for persistent problems and refer to the list when faced with new problems.
4. Remind your child of times when problems went away and better times followed.
5. Suggest the many positive ways the situation could turn out.
6. Join your child in his efforts to implement practical solutions.

---

her to recognize early when she may be heading into a downward spiral so she can talk herself out of it. Write down solutions to persistent problems and remind her to check them. Teach her that hardships will pass. If she has dorky glasses and people are teasing her about them, find better glasses. Help her find practical, positive solutions to her problems.

Therapy can be very helpful to you, too, if you feel overwhelmed by projecting your own fears and anxieties on the future. Teach yourself and your child to live one day at a time and that there's always tomorrow.

Live in the Now, but How?

The "now" word is for you! In some ways, bipolar disorder creates a secondary or reactionary bipolar disorder in parents. For example, as one parent said, "We all get exhausted and drained, which then creates tension and snippy behaviors among everyone in the house. Because no one is happy, everyone is miserable, and it turns into a vicious, unending cycle until someone accepts what is truly going on and assists the rest of the family to get back on board to support the child with bipolar disorder appropriately." You end up yelling and crying in frustration and feel like banging your head against the wall in desperation. You have to be "on" all the time—alert, neutral, appropriate, and compassionate—so that you can dish out positive feedback to your child. Then you reach a breaking point and you lose it. That is when living in the "now" can help you survive. Just focus on what is going on now and leave everything else for later. Tell yourself, "I am strong enough to cope. I can control my temper, and, if I can't, I will ask for help and find a friend or therapist or doctor to vent with." Practice this self-talk until you perfect it and it becomes second nature to let things that hurt you and push you to the limit roll off. This is "mindfulness."

Remember the journal I suggested you keep in Chapter 5? Make sure you take the opportunity to fill it with any inspiring mantras you run across that remind you to trust your own abilities. Keep it where you can reach it easily at any time, or transfer inspirational lines to a note card to keep in your wallet where you can pull them out to focus on when you're caught up in the heat of the moment. Whether we have a bipolar child in our life or not, we can all benefit from having a private source of strength like this. Not even the best therapist in the world knows as much about our situation and needs as we do. So lift ideas and phrases from personal growth books that inspire you and jot them down in your journal. When you have a problem, clarify your thinking using the "double column technique": make two columns on a page; then describe problems in one column and identify solutions in the other. I use a journal like this to inspire and guide my actions. I use it to center myself. For most of us, spirituality, peace, and positive thinking are not all that automatic, and we need to practice them with discipline. I write this part with sincerity and humility so you know that I practice what I preach and am not just telling you what to do!

Be a Good Friend: Building Social Skills

It is so important to help your child not only make friends but keep them. Many parents I've met resort to seeking out friends that seem suitable for their child after the child has lost many friends of his or her own choosing. You, too, may be tempted to do this when your child expresses loneliness and has no one to play with after school. But ask yourself how you would feel if someone chose a friend for you. Of course you want to protect your child from being hurt or led astray, but be sure to include friends your child actually *likes* among the possibilities you approve for play dates.

One reason you might want to act as your child's social "agent" is that you believe if you choose the right companion for your child you'll be able to set up a play date and the two of them will play by themselves. But you probably already know that's not likely to happen with a bipolar child, and it's not because your son or daughter hasn't been hanging around with the "right" kids. You need to continue to stick around and discreetly supervise playtime beyond the age that kids typically can be left to their own devices.

If this seems onerous (how are you going to get your work done and take care of other obligations with so little time available in your day?), remember that these are all "teaching moments." You can teach your bipolar child to treat peers with respect and learn the techniques of give and take that are important to healthy relationships. Be proactive in pulling your child out and teach appropriate skills if your child needs to be corrected on the spot. Be discreet and sensitive, but use those teaching moments. This is your chance to influence and shape your child one step at a time. I personally recommend choosing friends with parents who are likely to cooperate and, therefore, you feel less stressed about approaching. Make the process as easy as possible for yourself. Make a list of people you can comfortably call and enter them into your cell phone directory. Make a folder in your inbox to keep track of these parents' e-mails. Accept that it takes time to orchestrate these arrangements, but simplify the process as much as possible.

Balanced Lifestyle for You

"If I am not able to take care of myself in a good way, how can I show my daughter how to care for herself in a good way?"—a good question from one very wise parent. This practice is about finding time for you so there is balance in your life—otherwise, how will your child learn to find her own balance? Take a moment to draw a pie that shows what portion of your life is devoted to your bipolar child, your other children, partner, work, and finally yourself. I bet the portion for you is the smallest piece. While that is sad, you don't have to feel miserable. I, too, have a small pie for myself as I try to fit in everything I need to do, but my portion becomes bigger at times when I need to recharge my battery.

How do you recharge your battery? Are you able to take care of yourself and spend that energy and focus on *you*? Did you take that birthday off to indulge yourself? Do you get to do things you love once in a while? If you don't, list three things you like to do and make a point of finding time to do them. Don't say you don't have time. Even the CEOs of our largest corporations and our government leaders fit in golf and jogging. Keep it all in perspective, and be smart about taking care of yourself. If you don't

When you need to recharge, allow yourself a larger piece of the pie. It's only temporary and will model the importance of self-care for your child.

and bend over backward too much for others, you are doomed to fail. You need to show your child that you care enough to take time for yourself so your child learns healthy self-care habits for life. More ideas for taking good care of yourself are in Chapter 7.

Teaching Effective Problem Solving

It's important that you think like a manager, modeling effective problem-solving techniques and using persuasive influence rather than overt firmness to reduce reactivity in the bipolar child and yourself. Seeing the strengths in your child and figuring out how you and your child can solve problems collaboratively will get you through more crises than you can imagine. Treat your child with dignity and respect, like you would your good next-door neighbor. As I said, your respectful treatment will scaffold your child's self-esteem, but it also lays the necessary foundation for effective problem solving.

When problems erupt, one of the most important things to remember is not to touch the raging fire—that is, your child's explosive emotions—or you will get burned. Stay away until the tantrum dies down. Give the child space. Talk to your child when he is calm, perhaps when you kiss him good night. Describe the behavior you would like to see (specifying what ought to have happened earlier and what could be avoided) in a compassionate tone. It's hard to resist compassion. Also remember to get your child to apologize after a mishap. That allows your child to learn that she made a mistake and take responsibility for it.

It is critical that you do not withdraw privileges and mete out consequences in a standard behavior management way. Instead, we recommend approaching the problem using interpersonal psychotherapy-based problem-solving methods, rather than with standard behavior modification, which we know from experience will backfire with bipolar children. If your child has been diagnosed with ADHD, you may have already discovered that time-outs and points or other reward and punishment systems that can be helpful to kids with attention deficits and impulsivity just don't work well with your child. This does not mean, of course, that you're supposed to allow your child to behave in any way that strikes him (see "Ask–Say–Do" below), but imposing punishments per se is not going to be effective.

Behavior therapy is not recommended for bipolar children because they perceive punishment as a slight and start to distrust you, avoid you, get angry, and be irritable with you. It does not mean you should present your child with a new bike after he calls you a name, but you can say, "Well, it looks like things are tough right now. When you feel able to handle things and they start to go well, we will get you the new bike." This firm, determined message given with compassion will be more effective. It is the measured tone and timing that counts! Often, it is hard to stay calm and composed. I role-play with parents and you can practice if you like, imagining wearing a "robot hat," speaking in a neutral tone, and saying what you need to say with composure. At times, your child will hate your calmness, as he did not succeed in stirring you up. But, in the long run, if you practice staying calm and speaking steadily, the child will learn that he can't push you around. Complete silence from you can be seen as you neglecting him when he is trying to elicit a response from you. Give him attention by commenting briefly on how you will discuss the incident when you both are ready (like putting a comma but not a period on your conversation with him). Don't engage in long battles with the child in the middle of a storm. You are building bridges and need to get your child to trust you so he will follow your teachings and directions.

In my clinical practice, I model the dialogue between the parent and the bipolar child to demonstrate the best way to handle these conversations. The parent takes the role of the child, and I take the role of the parent. I ask the parents to challenge me as much as they want to, and I try to withstand the onslaught calmly. They often say it is easy for me to act appropriately for a short period in unreal situation. I disagree. In my experience, practice makes perfect—the more you practice dealing with these kids, the easier and more automatic it becomes. Here's an illustration:

Child: I want to go to the concert.

Parent: Who do you want to go with?

Child: With Alex, Tom, and Adrienne.

Parent: Well, I am not happy with the company, as I know they are into pot. Although I respect your choices, I feel it is my role to help you make the right decisions and choices. I am not happy about this one.

Child: Mom, I think you got it all wrong. I hate you. You are a moron, and I don't think you really care. All the respect you mention is fake. You just think I am wrong without knowing anything about my friends. Your friends are all hypocrites. What if I say you can't go out with them? [By this point, your child is panting and raving.]

Parent [speaking in a calm voice with a neutral tone and facial expression]: Honey, I know enough about what goes on and enough about these specific friends. I would not say the same about you going out with A.J., Ravi, and Jerry. If any one of them is going, I have no objection. I care about you. I said what I had to say. You think about it, darling. But I must say I feel sad when you call me a moron . . . [Put on slightly sad face and be matter-of-fact without raising your voice or showing anger]

At this point the child kicks the door. Even the family pet shivers and whimpers, and the tantrum becomes unbearable to watch. You then quietly withdraw from the conversation to show your unhappiness. Your child will eventually come and apologize (it could take a few minutes or a full day), recognizing that you care and were right and that she was nasty and should make amends. Stick to your guns, but gently, and don't readily try to please your child. Look sad and take your time to let her realize what she did. She will come back to you; you are too important to ignore!

Here is another example:

Parent: Larry, why don't you finish the project?

Child: I don't care. I don't have the proper pencil. I don't have the right material. My teacher is mean to give me the wrong U.S. state to write about.

Parent: Honey, it can be interesting to work on any state. How about we start collecting info? I will help with the pencil and how about . . . [Note that you did not yell back about the small issues, such as the complaints about the pencil or other materials, although you think it is a ridiculous excuse. You are respecting your child and getting him on your side by accommodating his mood a little bit.]

Child: [*intensely*] OK, then, but you have to search the computer yourself and get me the facts.

Parent: Of course I will help you, but how about if you open the computer and we both look? You are so good at this, you always amaze me . . . [Note that you did not immediately say, "No, you do it yourself. It is your project." Instead, you are in "yes mode" to get him on your side and gently steer him in the right direction as you release yourself from doing all of it. Situations like this can easily explode, but, recognizing that bipolar children have difficulty making the transition to homework, it is wiser to negotiate than fight. By saying yes, you get your child to do it all

---

Gain Cooperation Using Ask–Say–Do

Note: *This is a simple technique that can be used with children under age 10 or so. But I caution against using it when your child is raging or "hyped up."*

"**Ask–Say–Do**" can help reduce oppositionality in the younger bipolar child. Here's how it works: **Ask,** "Can you do this, please?" If there's no response, then **Say,** "Do this now." If that doesn't get results, then **Do** by physically intervening to make your child do what you are asking. For example: **Ask:** "Please brush your teeth, Tom." **Say:** "Brush your teeth." **Do:** Escort Tom by the arm to the sink to make him brush with minimal fuss. This technique tells your child that you mean business and are in control of the situation, but in order for it to work you need to be fully involved and committed to following through. Leave no room for negotiations or boundary pushing. Unequivocal expectation from you will gently teach your child to cooperate. If there's a tantrum, explosion, or rage, give it time to run its course. Of course, there are times you will fail and things will fall apart. You must pick up the thread again at the next opportunity. Review what happened when your child is calm. Give her a pep talk about what happened and how it could have gone differently. Each time you do it, you reinforce the message that your child must cooperate with your expectations.

in the end. If your child goes into a rage anyway, you can do little at that moment. Let go of the situation and try again when your child is calm and ready to talk.]

Remember: It takes longer and causes a lot more heartache if you feel aggravated. Take it easy and practice these skills.

Ways to Get Support

Bipolar disorder can be isolating, both for the child who has it and for other family members, who may feel shame or discomfort talking about their situation. Therapy can help children and parents get past their fears, identify reliable sources of support, and encourage them to reach out to their network in times of crisis. Professionals, such as doctors, nurses, and social workers, can become ongoing sources of support. Joining a support group can help you feel like you aren't alone. "I hear other people who have gone through some of the same stuff," a parent said. "I learned from how they handled their situations."

When cultivating and maintaining sources of support gets stale, therapy can encourage both the child and parents to reconnect to keep their network alive. Draw a tree with branches and roots to represent your support system. Who can you go to in crisis? Who can serve as a mentor? Who is available for play dates? For holidays? For hanging out? To get tutoring? To play catch? Who are the best choices at school? At Boy Scouts? In the neighborhood? At your church, synagogue, temple, or mosque? Who is available and of practical value?

Don't forget to create a support tree for yourself, too! Know who is in the inner circle. Who is in the next circle? Figure out how to get support from a variety of places so you won't burn out your resources and tire out your precious best friend.

What If I Can't Find CFF-CBT–Based Therapy for My Bipolar Child?

As expert care and therapy is not always accessible, in some situations you may not have access to the full range of therapeutic expertise that is best for the bipolar child. You and your doctor may need to piece together a program using the best available options in your area. Some therapy is better than no therapy at all, and you might need to adapt different therapeutic programs to touch on the key principles of CFF-CBT–based RAINBOW therapy as I have outlined it throughout this chapter. More important than the type of therapy is finding a practitioner who specializes or has substantial experience in treating bipolar disorder in children. A lot depends on the capabilities and willingness of the therapist to incorporate the concepts we have been discussing, but you can also employ these strategies by yourself at home. That said, there are two types of therapy to avoid definitely:

- Behavior therapy: As I said earlier, straightforward unmodified behavior therapy is *not* recommended for children with bipolar disorder. Indeed, many of the techniques that work for typical kids (or even those with ADHD), such as establishing a routine and rewarding positive behavior, can be helpful with the bipolar child. But others, such as enforcing consequences, can backfire horribly. You need a therapy that directly addresses your child's severe mood swings and that does not provoke negative feelings and thoughts. As I've said, these children are highly rejection sensitive. Dozens of books have been written on behavior management, most of which offer sound advice for the vast majority of families, but negative consequences "without frills" may not apply for bipolar kids. It's very important to apply behavior management techniques judiciously and appropriately given the volatile and sensitive nature of the bipolar child.
- Play therapy is generally not harmful, but it does not teach parents how to cope with severe mood swings or discipline an unwieldy bipolar child. I feel it is inappropriate for parents to drop off kids for hour-long therapy appointments and not have a chance to learn the skills necessary to cope with these kids. Explore your doctor's or therapist's philosophy of treatment and get lots of tips for managing your child. Learning the ropes from the therapist on how to coach your child is equal to or more important than the therapist's direct work with the child. Effective therapy for your child has to include a direct, active parent component.

Phases of Treatment

CFF-CBT for childhood bipolar disorder includes sessions for parents alone, children alone, and the family together, with an emphasis on individual psychotherapy with children, parent training and support, and family therapy. The intensity and timing of this treatment program, as well as which members of the family are involved, can change over time as your child progresses from one stage or "phase" of treatment to another.

Acute Phase

For the first 6 months, when your doctor is still trying to get your child's symptoms under control, you might have frequent sessions, up to once a week. Under the RAINBOW protocol, we usually recommend no fewer than 12 sessions, focusing on seven core ingredients (routine, affect or mood regulation, self-esteem, positive thinking, social skill building, interpersonal problem solving, and social support) over a 6- to 9-month period.

Maintenance Phase

As I mentioned before, bipolar disorder is a lifelong illness that changes as your child grows and develops. Therefore, maintenance treatment is very important. The number and frequency of sessions will vary between every 2 weeks or once a month to twice a year, depending on how well your child is doing and your family's access to the clinic. Again, our own research following bipolar children over a 3-year period after receiving initial therapy showed that maintenance sessions did sustain recovery. A maintenance program that follows the principles outlined in this chapter, combined with medication, can reduce the potential for relapse and helps sustain positive changes over time. This takes the form of booster sessions. Our research indicates that during the maintenance phase booster sessions may be needed to overcome specific issues that tend to crop up over time, for instance, defiance that lingers for a long time, regressing from following a basic routine, uncontrolled aggression or excitability, isolation, withdrawal, feeling helpless or hopeless, lying and risk taking, continued academic struggles, grandiosity or bossiness, feeling teased or scapegoated, parents being overwhelmed or overextended, and increased conflict at home or at school. Various intervention strategies, designed to reestablish the basic principles of CFF-CBT, are introduced to offset difficult behaviors, reinforce positive thinking and problem solving, and reinvigorate parents' commitment. For instance, if your child continues to struggle socially, the therapist might suggest that you focus on a small circle of positive friendships. If you are starting to feel like your child is fight-

---

A Typical RAINBOW Timetable

To stabilize your child's moods: We usually expect it to take 4–9 months for medication and therapy to stabilize your child's moods—doctor's visits every 3–4 weeks during the first 4–6 months (or however long it takes to find an effective combination of medications), along with CFF-CBT therapy sessions at least twice a month (at least 12 sessions) for up to 9 months.

To stay on track and respond to changes: Maintenance CFF-CBT therapy sessions anywhere from twice a month to twice a year, as needed. They serve as booster sessions to address specific issues, and doctor's visits should serve to adjust medication as needed.

---

ing a losing battle, the therapist might provide a pep talk and validate the success you've already achieved. However, there are no magic solutions that will fix these problems instantly. It is important to revisit the techniques above and rejuvenate your enthusiasm and efforts to pull yourself together and start again. You can do it.

Where to Get Therapy for Your Child

Professional Assistance

Your doctors' qualifications and background, along with your insurance coverage, will help determine the type of therapy and the location in which it will take place. As I discussed in Chapter 3, a child psychiatrist with experience in bipolar disorder is the linchpin of your treatment program—he or she will be able to provide state-of-the-art medication management and make sure your child receives the integrated, coordinated psychosocial support described earlier in this chapter.

Unfortunately, in many situations, a well-prepared specialist is not available and you might have to piece together a team. Most of the time, the team will be based on your doctor's recommendations, although asking other parents in the same situation can be very helpful. Many parents shy away from waiting lists, but it is frequently worth the wait. Be a little patient. Don't shop and change medications in desperation or fire a good doctor if you can help it just based on limited availability. Resources are limited, and qualified specialists are stretched thin. My advice is to hang in there and work with the best clinician you can.

Keep in mind that your insurance plan may also influence the therapy program. In general, therapy is delivered by one or more of the following:

- Clinical psychologist: a PhD or PsyD child psychologist with experience with bipolar disorder is preferable to a general child or adult psychologist. A psychologist can generally provide the full range of therapy but will need to work with your doctor on medication management.
- Social worker: a master's or PhD-level social worker can provide social support and therapy and help you deal with the school if your primary doctor lacks expertise in this area. A licensed clinical social worker (LCSW) also has advanced clinical experience that may be beneficial to your family.
- Therapist: This term covers a range of professionals with backgrounds in social work, psychology, counseling, nursing, or education having an advanced degree and/or licensure in various treatment approaches. When evaluating whether to work with a particular therapist, give preference to someone experienced in bipolar disorder and related family dynamics.

Treatment Locations

Therapy can be delivered in a number of settings, depending on the child's symptoms, stage of treatment, and other circumstances. Again, insurance plans may influence when, where, and how often your child can be treated, but in general:

- During the acute phase, your child might have to be admitted to a hospital or residential treatment program to be stabilized. If there's a relapse or other episode, she might have to be readmitted for a medication adjustment and/or a therapy booster. Severely affected children—those who are a danger to themselves or others around them—require longer-term institutionalization, for instance in a special hospital or residential treatment center. See Chapter 9 for more information on away-from-home placement.
- For less severe symptoms, an outpatient clinic or therapist's office

What Are Your Options in a Crisis?

Most families never have to experience a psychiatric hospitalization for their child or find a residential treatment facility, but some do. Because of the nature of the illness and the safety concerns that frequently accompany bipolar symptoms, more restrictive types of service can be necessary. There are varied levels of crises; what may seem like a crisis today may not feel that way tomorrow. However, if your child cannot be safely maintained at home or is having unremitting or unusually intense difficulties at home or school, you may need to consider one of the following options:

- **Hospitalization:** This may involve having your child spend a few days to several weeks in a hospital psychiatric unit or youth facility. This is generally a short-term strategy designed to get an acute situation under control, especially when a child needs round-the-clock supervision or close monitoring. Hospitalization is also helpful when making a major medication change or introducing a new therapy, with the goal of returning the child to his own home and regular school once the crisis ends. Families tell us that they have checked into providers in their area, asked other families about their experiences, and investigated coverage when their child's moods were stable. Knowing in advance about coverage also helps families and mental health providers know when to use benefits or save them.
- **Residential treatment centers (RTCs):** RTCs are secure facilities designed for children with extensive clinical and educational needs who cannot be safely maintained at home. According to the National Association of Therapeutic Schools and Programs (NATSAP), most of these centers are Joint Commission on Accreditation of Healthcare Organizations (JCAHO) accredited. They manage and monitor children's medication, hold group and individual therapy sessions, and schedule recreational activities along with academic programs. Centers vary widely in size; you may find the smaller ones with more specific areas of focus more appealing than the larger facilities, but weighing your child's needs and the offerings of available facilities can be a complicated matter. Fortunately, the NATSAP website (*www.natsap.org*) is packed with useful information, advice, and resources and may be a great relief to read. The association recommends that if you're considering placing your child in a residential center for a time, you obtain the help of a consultant to identify the best setting for your child.
- Also see the discussion of therapeutic day schools in Chapter 9.

is preferable. Outpatient treatment can be more or less intensive depending on the need. In a crisis, you might have three or four sessions a week, while in the maintenance phase, visits could be weekly or even less frequent.

- Some programs can provide therapy at home or school if the situation warrants it. You will have to do some research with local agencies and healthcare providers to find these programs. This can be an ideal way to offer real-world assistance with behavior management or educate family members, teachers, and others who interact with your child on a regular basis.

Getting Help for the Whole Family

Parents, siblings, and other family members have needs that may extend beyond the scope of CFF-CBT. In that case, supportive psychotherapy may be used to help the child and family through difficult and stressful situations by offering empathy and support as they address their problems. Some sources of additional support include:

- For yourself: If you are particularly stressed, burned out, or depressed, talk it over candidly with your doctor. It is very hard to expect you to be up to doing things well with your child if you are not in a good mental state. Even if you are not the cause of the problem or not seriously ill, therapy can put things in perspective for you. I will give you more ideas for taking care of yourself in Chapter 7.
- For you and your spouse: Sometimes a pastor, priest, or rabbi can do this if you both are of the same religious persuasion. Also, professionally trained and licensed marriage counselors are available in pretty much every locale. Sometimes it may be something a social worker, psychologist, or psychiatrist does, but you'll have to ask around. Check with your doctor, who will likely know a few names. As with family therapy, don't go into this blind. Find someone you both can trust. Talk with friends who have been through marriage counseling, and see if there is anyone they can recommend. It can be stressful, but if the relationship is in a tailspin, don't wait until it is too late to recover.

Is *Your* Emotional Health Getting in the Way of Your Managing Your Child's Condition?

Ask yourself these questions:

- Are you struggling with depression, ADHD, bipolar disorder, or another mental illness? If so, your child's symptoms may look normal to you, making it hard for you to recognize a problem in your child and causing you to delay seeking help for him or her.
- Do your mood swings tax your patience for dealing with your child?
- If your illness were treated, would your child do better? One parent said, "As a result of my daughter's diagnosis, I was forced to take a hard look at my own background—I was tested as an adult (39 years old), and I have bipolar disorder myself. The treatment plan developed for myself has had a positive impact on my relationships with my husband and daughters."

If you think your mental health is getting in the way of helping your child, talk to your doctor about starting treatment. Many parents dealing with this difficult disorder receive medication and therapy for anxiety, depression, and other symptoms that may be a by-product of living with a child with bipolar disorder. You owe it to yourself and your child to get treatment.

- For a sibling or other member of the family: When a sibling is tormented by a child with bipolar disorder and watches conflict develop between parents because of that child's bipolar disorder, troublesome feelings about the bipolar child can definitely develop. How are kids supposed to handle these uncomfortable feelings, especially when Mom and Dad are simply too busy to take charge? As one parent pointed out ruefully, "Health insurance does not pay for counseling for the other kids." In fact, almost all insurance companies will pay for what are called "collateral visits," where other family members can be seen as a means of assisting the primary patient. In addition, if parents and/or siblings have their own difficulties, there will be similar coverage within that insurance program for each family member, based on each of them receiving his or her own diagnosis.

The Most Important Ingredient Is You

As you've probably gathered already, I believe that parents are a pretty important part of the child's recovery! The tone you set at home, the way you handle ups and downs at school, and how you manage to get what your child needs make an enormous difference in how your child fares, and that's what the RAINBOW approach is intended to help you do. In the next chapter, I'll talk more about how you can maintain your equilibrium, keep your poise under duress, and be the best possible advocate for your child, yourself, and the rest of your family. You can do this!

SEVEN

Parenting with Poise

THE SECRET INGREDIENT
FOR SUCCESS

"One of the challenges of living with a bipolar child is the daily need for teaching/modeling behavior management at a much higher level than needed for a 'typical' child."

As parents, you are the single most important support and anchor for your child, the secret ingredient for success in treating childhood bipolar disorder. Although it seems tempting to let go and let the doctors and hospitals take over, it rarely works out that way—and it shouldn't. You are your child's first and best advocate, the one who knows her ups and downs, the one who understands her daily challenges, her friends and social environment, and the strengths and limitations of your family, school system, and community.

I know it sounds like a pretty demanding and at times overwhelming job. However, you *can* maintain your poise and confidence, even when things have taken a difficult turn. In order to do so, you must understand the limits of what you can accomplish, let go of the things you cannot control, and know how to keep yourself energized, not just for your child, but also for yourself.

Dealing with Your Own Feelings

Parents tell us that one of the hardest parts of bipolar disorder is fully accepting their child as he is, while helping him to be responsible for his behavior. Parents who reach this stage say that they are able to applaud their child's uniqueness and actually view it as a gift or blessing. You need to believe that your child can have a bright and happy future, despite the many obstacles standing in his way. As one parent put it, "Your child's brain is wired differently. Love her for who she is, not what you thought she would be."

I have seen supportive, gentle guidance from parents make a tremendous difference. I compare the progress children make with this guidance to that of growing taller. Can you see your child grow taller each day? No. But you can tell the difference from season to season or year to year. Your son's or daughter's emotional maturity and perspective will also grow slowly over time if there is stable treatment coupled with the right kind of support from you.

It takes constant vigilance as a parent to deal with your own feelings toward your child. A certain amount of resentment and anger is normal. Sometimes you cannot help but react to a crisis and say the wrong thing in the heat of the moment. You are, after all, a human being with your own emotions, and your child's mood swings inevitably will trigger a variety of reactions, including fear, anger, frustration, and despair. There are going to be disappointments and failures, but it is important that you don't pass those feelings along to your child. As much as possible, you need to act like a dam that stops the flood of feelings. You carry an extra burden, without a doubt! There are no shortcuts, and you must be the stronger one here, but by reading this book you have taken an important step to prepare yourself with the skills you need to cope.

Always remember, your child can't help having this disease. He cannot "snap out of it." Understand his limitations, but help him find areas where he can excel. Help him understand his moods without allowing him to use them as an excuse to hurt others or himself. It's a very fine line to walk. In order to do so, it is important to comprehend the nature of the disorder. The RAINBOW strategies described in Chapter 6 are designed to help you and your child work together to solve the problems imposed by bipolar disorder while remaining positive and optimistic about what each of you can achieve.

Often, bipolar children will insist on their view and push relentlessly, without yielding to logic. Suddenly, your child who is capable of normal logic sounds insane and you feel exasperated. That is when you should use the powerful technique of "diverting attention." Forget about the issue at hand and try to amuse her, ask a question in a matter-of-fact manner on some other topic, show her something, or tell her what happened yesterday at the fair. Wisdom, not logic, is your savior. Understand that **your goal is not to prove to your child that you are right—your goal is managing your child!** You will see how quickly she can be managed through the technique of diversion.

Of course, life is uncertain, more complicated, and much messier than we would like. Even if you try very hard to create a stable, nurturing home life, you still will need to cope with the unexpected. Bipolar disorder is unpredictable by definition. It is cyclical, chronic, and strikes in different ways at different times, so what worked last year (or even last month) may not work today. Knowing this may put you on edge, waiting for the event that upsets the apple cart. It may make you feel like you're walking on eggshells. This is when you should think, "I will take it one step at a time. Today, I will focus on. . . . This is all one can do in this situation." Be your own wise monk.

Who can you talk to at these times? It can be hard to find others who care, and even when you do, they don't know enough of the details to be helpful. So you will need to find a center of gravity in yourself. Sometimes, a sense of humor and talk with a close friend will help ease the pain. Sometimes, just writing in a journal will help you come up with solutions to difficult problems. Ironically, when we reach "the right place" inside ourselves as parents, we can embrace the unpredictability and even come to see it as an interesting part of the disorder.

Bringing Out the Best in Your Child

No matter how hard it is for you to cope with this changeable, invisible brain disorder, imagine how hard it is for your child. Bipolar children must learn to love and accept themselves, which is a much harder task for them than for their parents. Compassion is the magic ingredient. As I said earlier, children with bipolar disorder are supersensitive and vulnerable to criticism. Their self-esteem is very fragile. "No matter how upset you are with their behavior, try not to communicate that you are disappointed in who they are," one parent said. "Rather, teach them to accept themselves and arm them with knowledge." Another parent suggests, "Just love your child. Take numerous deep breaths a day and remember it's *not* their fault (or yours). Helping them find ways to succeed will be the key."

Knowing what is going on in your child's world will greatly enhance your ability to experience life through his eyes. It's no fun getting frustrated and angry at small things, being excitable, or irritating others (even you). Your bipolar child often feels alone despite his desire to be the center of attention. He can be bubbly and ebullient, yet shunned by his peers and seen as a problem child by teachers. He tries hard to connect with others, only to alienate them with his bossiness and intensity. Feeling sad and trying to hide it is a daily struggle. If understanding this doesn't make you feel compassionate, what will? One of my mentors said, if you can't hug your child physically, you can "hug with your eyes"—showing lots of love and compassion in your gaze.

When your child is having a meltdown, it is tempting to call your doctor seeking a "magic bullet"—a new medication, treatment technique, or behavioral tool—then get irritated that it didn't fix the problem. Keeping in touch with clinicians, getting their advice, and alerting them to a poor response to medications is part and parcel of helping your child. But often the problem isn't bipolar-related, and there is no quick fix. Occasionally, stressful events in life trigger dysfunctional behavior in children that may appear to be a mood swing, but is *not* bipolar disorder. A careful analysis will help you distinguish symptoms of bipolar disorder from reactions to medication changes or emotional turmoil that has nothing to do with bipolar disorder.

At times like these, what your child really may need is A *DOSE OF YOU*—that is, more parental time and attention, rather than a new medication or therapist. This may interfere with your schedule or take time away from your other children, but you may need to do it anyway. Your attention will help build a trust and love that speak volumes. If you don't know what to say, hang out and play or just be together. This will help satisfy your child's seemingly bottomless neediness, at least for the time being, building bridges and intimacy slowly but surely.

Your child needs your help dealing with the confusing, sometimes paralyzing transitions between acceptance and encouragement at home and rejection and discouragement everywhere else. An enlightened parent is perhaps the only one who can counteract the damage to self-esteem that occurs when the outside world treats the bipolar child cruelly (as it will). Your job is to be their anchor in the storm. "My child was passed from teacher to teacher," relates one parent, "and just when he bonded with one, he'd be moved to a different classroom. He took it as not being liked anymore. It is very difficult to maintain a child's self-esteem when he gets passed like a ball from place to place." Just imagine being in this child's shoes. It is hard enough to move once; imagine how hard it is to move a lot *and* be criticized, while coping with a serious illness. It's not a double whammy, but a triple whammy!

An attitude of acceptance and understanding—without excuses—is the very hallmark of love for a child, a love remarkable for its resilience and endurance despite all you go through as a parent. I bet you could feel this from the very beginning. At times, it is hard to stay so noble and loving, and it may help to model yourself on a person you admire or look up to, or even a TV or movie character. Find the strength to stay calm and be a rock that your child can lean on. Act the part when everything is falling to pieces until you are able to integrate this strength into your regular behavior.

Help Your Child Understand the Disorder

Hard as it may be to believe, honesty is the best policy when it comes to telling your child about bipolar disorder. In fact, if you try to hide the truth, your child is more likely to think she's "bad"—that this is her fault—and her self-esteem will plummet. For instance, some parents want their child to wait outside while they are telling me their problems. While that is perfectly fine, and I respect their wishes, I often tell them that it is okay to discuss the subject in front of their child if they do it in a respectful, gentle manner.

It is much more beneficial to teach bipolar children about their disorder, explain that their brains are wired differently, and offer them ways to cope. Explaining the science can help them understand that it really isn't their fault. Give them the information in small pieces, so they aren't confused or overwhelmed. Yes, your child's disorder makes him different, but remind him that he is much more than his disorder and that he needn't define himself based on his mood swings. He is a unique person with his own personality, talents, and abilities, different from but no less special than his brothers, sisters, or other children he knows. It might help him to know that he may not have the disorder forever—like many others, he could potentially outgrow it or learn to live with it effortlessly.

Despite your reassurances, your child might still feel alone and isolated. It can be comforting to know about other loved family members or even celebrities your child looks up to who have triumphed over bipolar disease—like actors Jim Carrey and Ben Stiller, musicians Sting and for-

Explaining Bipolar Disorder to Your Child

Look for occasions and opportunities to teach your child about bipolar disorder in a way that helps him understand what is going on in his brain (how it affects his thoughts and behavior) and reassures him that he is not to blame. Remember to do this when your child is calm (not in the middle of an outburst or meltdown) and better able to process the information you are imparting.

Parent: Now that you feel all right [approach the child when he is really feeling good, not just a bit better], do you think we can talk about what was hard for us?

Child: No.

Parent: Well, we have to, sweetie. It was tough for you when I said that was enough TV. Can you tell me what made you so mad? [Notice that I am avoiding asking "Why?" and using "What?" instead.]

Child: I don't know. Sometimes my brain just makes me scream. It is not me.

Parent: I can tell that these mad feelings came over you like a blanket and you could not help it at that time. Right, darling? [Notice that here I am using kind words, but I suggest that you be clear and firm and not sickly sweet.]

Child: Is something wrong with my brain?

Parent: Your brain is just fine, sweetie. But there are strengths and weaknesses for everybody. Perhaps your brain is a tad bit more reactive to anything you see as a criticism or when you don't like something. It's not your fault, but you can learn to train it. How your brain is wired causes you to explode perhaps, but there are fantastic ways to learn to control these emotions. You can tame your brain and cool it off when you are mad or hyped up!

Child: How? That is impossible to do. I don't even know I get like that.

Parent: Hey, hey, you can—I know you can. We need to understand your moods and figure out what color your mood is in if you are starting to feel uncomfortable. If you see you're going into the red zone, stop and think before you act. Trust me, with time it gets so easy, like second nature *and you can do it!* You can only try, right? Can you tell me one example when you were able to stop?

Child: OK, I remember the time when I stopped. . . . [If you are lucky, you will get an example to begin to reflect on.]

Parent: I know you can. The more you think about it and the more you know about it, the better it will be for you!

Focus on age-appropriate information: Imagine the same conversation with children of different ages. You may want to avoid that "talking to a child" tone with older kids and sound more mature in discussions with them. You just need to know that you can debrief your child after an incident, helping her retrace her steps. Sometimes, just listening to the child talk about how she could not control herself is productive, without preaching. You are listening, which is very, very powerful!

mer Beach Boy Brian Wilson, or athletes like tennis star Ilie Nastase and football player Alonzo Spellman. Explain how bipolar disorder can make people more sensitive to others' needs or enhance their creativity. More important, highlight the healthy aspects of your child's personality and identify positive traits, such as persistence or enthusiasm—things he can take ownership of that have nothing to do with bipolar disorder.

On the other hand, don't dwell on bipolar disorder all the time. Your child needs to remember that bipolar disorder is something apart from him as a person, so treat it in the same way as you would a child's need for eyeglasses (although, certainly, this is a much bigger intrusion on the

You Can Be a Positive Bipolar Role Model

If you or someone else close to your child has overcome bipolar disorder or another mental illness, you may or may not choose to share this information, but if there's been an official diagnosis, everyone may already know. When your child reaches an age where he or she can understand, sit down and tell your story. Explain how you found out you had the disorder, and describe what you do to deal with it (take medications, go to therapy, practice problem-solving techniques, etc.). When similar situations come up for your child, explain that you often feel/felt the same way and explain how you cope. Your child will not only see that he is not alone, he'll learn from your good example! Hopefully, it will drive home the message to your child that it is not his fault and someone close to him may have the same struggles he has!

child's life): identify role models with glasses, teach your child how to live with glasses, and leave it at that. Don't rub it in.

Since bipolar disorder runs in families, it is possible that some family members have fared less well with the disease. Be honest with your child about the challenges these relatives face, but reassure her that these problems aren't inevitable for her—not with the love and support of a strong and committed family like yours. Guilt and self-blame are very destructive emotions, whether in you or your child. It is much more helpful and productive to take a problem-solving attitude: candidly and openly admitting and accepting the disease, fixing what can be fixed, and moving forward. You want to model this behavior and encourage the same in your child. Tell her about how you coped with your problems, without getting melodramatic, as a way to give her courage and hope. Don't sweat it; it is hard for all of us as parents not to feel guilty for one thing or another about our children, especially these children.

Accentuate the Positive

As I said earlier in this book, because bipolar kids are sensitive and volatile, it is best to emphasize the positive and downplay the negative. Behavioral techniques that work on average children can backfire. Punishment and consequences can create unnecessary power struggles that are exhausting and counterproductive.

Use your ingenuity to find good things in your child. This is what I tell parents when they give up and say there is nothing positive to report. In therapy, we tell children to write out all their good experiences and stories of how they are/were winners. Read them. Add to them based on your observations. Embrace them. Teach your children how to say good things about themselves using that positive inner voice. Load their positive inner voice with statements about how good they are and use those thoughts to scaffold their confidence. Build self-esteem through positive storytelling. Tell them, "You can do this." This is so simple, yet so central.

Help your child think of solutions to negative thoughts. It could start with you reframing the harsh thoughts the child might have about herself. Help her think of how to change unhelpful thoughts or experiences to helpful ones. She needs to minimize catastrophic thinking, learn not to make mountains out of molehills, and keep things in perspective. As you work through these issues with your child, you will also learn to use these

Turning Negative Thoughts into Positive Ones

Negative Thought	Positive Alternative
I never do anything right.	Everybody makes mistakes. I'll learn from this and try again.
Nobody likes me.	Nobody is liked by everyone. I will focus on what is good about me and others. I have quite a few good friends I can call on.
I always lose, so why try?	This situation will pass, and I will feel good again.
These bad feelings will never end.	**I do not need to mope.** I'll let it roll right off me, like water off a duck's back.

strategies yourself. There will be no more looking through dark goggles for either of you. You can start to live in the now and not overwhelm yourself with questions like "What's next?" or "Will rage rip me apart again soon?"

Cultivate Strengths and Talents

As I mentioned earlier, all children have islands of competence, strengths and talents that promote confidence and self-esteem. In fact, bipolar children may exhibit many above-average capabilities, such as creativity, verbal abilities, and high energy, that make them stand out in many areas.

The best place to begin cultivating your child's strengths is by exploring activities that she likes to do, whether drama, art, music, sports, or something else. Drama can be an especially good outlet for bipolar children's grandiosity, letting them take center stage and express themselves verbally. When it comes to sports, individual sports such as tennis are easier to find partners for than team sports. Swimming can help these intense children expend pent-up energy and be more relaxed.

There may be times when you will need to look for special programs. You can talk to coaches or camp directors, or even get a letter from a doctor or therapist to reassure them that your child is suitable and provide ideas for helping your child function in the program. For example, I wrote a letter to Disney World for special accommodations for a bipolar child. Remember that coaches or supervisors are not always as savvy and sophisticated as healthcare professionals. Give them information, but don't make such a fuss that they get hypervigilant and call too much attention to your child's needs.

Your bipolar child may change his mind constantly. Encourage him to stick with an interest long enough to develop a skill. If he doesn't, he won't develop the competence that leads to enjoyment or even a passion for an activity. Consider yourself extremely lucky if your child finds his passion.

Enhance Resilience

Because they tend to generalize from negative experiences and project these generalizations into the future, bipolar children are easily disappointed and see themselves as failures. You can help your child build resilience by reminding her frequently that everyone loses out sometimes and that challenges are a part of life. Teach your child some comforting statements to make to herself when things don't go as planned, such as "If at first you don't succeed, try, try again," or "It's not whether you win or lose; it's how you play the game." Demonstrating your resilience, such as explaining how you regained a positive outlook after a particularly trying period, can also be very helpful.

Your child's generally negative outlook can even intrude on what should be happy times. These children may climb to the top of a mountain and still feel dissatisfied. You can help your child understand that there is no magic way to create a peak experience. When older, your child may engage in high-risk behavior just for the thrill. It is important to teach him to live in the moment and enjoy reality without exaggerated expectations or unattainable dreams. We can all learn to be content with what we have—it isn't just a problem with bipolar children, although it is often an issue with them.

Advocating for Your Child

Being your child's main advocate can seem pretty overwhelming, particularly when you must challenge doctors, hospitals, insurance companies, and school systems to make sure that your child gets exactly what she needs.

The Healthcare System

These days most people view doctors less as experts and more as consultants who know illness and child development, advising the family, who knows the child best. This is a change from an earlier era, in which doctors were viewed as absolute authority figures. Some doctors are uncomfortable having their recommendations questioned or taking suggestions from family members or other practitioners. Some patients may even have difficulty asking probing questions or insisting on a particular treatment approach for their child for fear of appearing disrespectful. You (or your insurance company, which you pay via premiums) pay the doctor's salary, so, in a real sense, she does work for you. See the doctor as your partner. Genuine questions asked in a genuine way will generally serve you well.

This does not mean that you should act entitled or take an attitude of "the customer is always right," but in the long run you have to be comfortable with your relationships with your child's doctor; you need to "find a good doctor that you click with," as one parent put it. As your ultimate goal is to get your child the help he needs, you need to make sure you're getting help and advice from the doctor. If not, it's important to work these issues out. Seek another opinion, or find another doctor. "You have to take great care in selecting the professionals you need," is the way one parent put it. "Then you need to listen to them and trust them—until you have good reason not to."

It is important that you respect your physician's training and experience, but that doesn't mean keeping your questions and concerns to yourself. Your child's well-being is ultimately your responsibility, and it's important that you advocate for his or her needs and those of the rest of the family. As I discussed in Chapter 3, you play such an important role in the management of your child's treatment that you must stay in the decision-making loop. Establishing a partnership with your doctor, combined with ongoing discussion, problem solving, and sharing of opinions and concerns among all members of the care team, both professional and lay, is a necessary part of that process.

The School System

It also can be hard to steel yourself to take on a large and complex institution like the schools. You may be weary and feel like you've already fought far too many wars—with the healthcare system, with well-meaning family members, maybe even with your spouse—just to get a correct diagnosis for your child. Despite your fatigue, it is very important that you approach the schools in a calm, neutral, and businesslike manner. Dress nicely and maintain your poise, even if you're feeling less than confident to start with. It can be nice to bring food—meetings often take place during lunch or planning hours or before school, and school staff may not have had time to eat. There can be many delays, obstacles, and hurdles to get over, so save your energy and don't overreact. It will just hurt your case. Taking an experienced parent with you who can support you in negotiating with the school can make a big difference here. Another parent can not only help articulate your child's needs, but also can give you the moral support and understanding you need to carry on. Also, there's no reason to assume that you're going to have a battle with the school system, despite what you may have heard or read elsewhere. Start out thinking positively and you might be pleasantly surprised.

After all, every state has laws to define and protect the rights of parents in special education processes. You find out about them by linking to your state's Parent–Teacher Associations (PTA) via *www.pta.org*. The Bazelon Center also provides a list of state parent advocacy links at *www.bazelon.org/links/states/index.htm*, or you can go directly to the website of your state's Parent Training and Information Centers and Community Parent Resource Centers (*www.taalliance.org/centers/index.htm*). which are federally funded to serve families of children and young adults with disabilities from birth to age 22.

There are also many independent parent support and advocacy groups that offer printed material, web-based resources, workshops, and phone consultation. The Child and Adolescent Bipolar Foundation (CABF) and the Learning Disabilities Association of America are two good places to start. See the Resources for more. In the final analysis, there's no substitute for experience, so if you can team up with an experienced parent who has done it before, it can save you a lot of time and give you the moral and practical support you need. You might even want to take this parent-mentor along to your meetings with the school staff should you request special education or special accommodations within the general education setting for your child. Your doctor may be able to match you with another experienced parent, or you can search on the Internet through CABF or another parent support group.

To obtain legal representation, contact the protection and advocacy system in your state via the National Disability Rights Network (*www.napas.org*). Alternatively, you might contact the Commission on Mental and Physical Disability Law (CMPDL) at *www.abanet.org/disability*. You may also find other agencies in your state on the Bazelon Center website's list of state advocacy links.

Chapter 9 goes into great detail about how to work successfully with the school system to meet your bipolar child's educational needs.

Taking Care of Yourself

"I had to learn to find things to enjoy again such as gardening and writing. I've tried to enjoy little things like a cup of tea or a few moments to sit outside on a swing. Taking a few quick moments to renew oneself can make all the difference in the world."

"I can't solve all of my son's problems and I've been learning not to feel guilty about that. I've put everything in place that is within my power. The rest is prayer and a power bigger than me. What a load that was off my mind to let go of feeling responsible for trying to make everything perfect."

What about you? How can you maintain your poise and persevere when your home life is constantly in flux? How can you model a balanced lifestyle when dealing with your child takes up so much of your energy? How can you continue to advocate for your child if you do end up facing opposition from the healthcare system, school district, or insurance company? How do you accomplish all this without becoming stressed or depressed yourself? The only way is by taking the time to take care of yourself.

At this point you're probably saying to yourself, "Take care of myself? Who has time, when managing my child and household, not to mention trying to hold a job, is a 24-7 commitment?" This is absolutely true, but I am challenging you to find a way to do it. Unload some responsibilities; let things around the house go a little; find respite care or a great babysitter; do whatever it takes to take a few precious minutes to rest and recharge your spirit. Chapter 8 includes many more ideas for streamlining and simplifying your life to find the time you need to make your home life smoother. Many of those strategies will help you take care of yourself as well.

In many ways, taking care of yourself is central to everything you do.

It is like driving a car. You need to fill the car with gas to make it go. You need to maintain the engine and other parts to keep the car performing at its peak. You are like the car—you need fuel, maintenance, and repair to keep going. Otherwise, you will run out of gas.

You will be happier and more relaxed if you feel good about yourself. And the happier you are, the more you will be able to respond to others, including your bipolar child, when the chips are down. When we feel overstressed and irritable—something that happens to all of us—our tempers flare, and we may end up doing or saying things that we regret. This is a part of life, but it is a part of life we want to minimize if possible, as it tends to make things worse and add to our other burdens and challenges.

Think of your mind as a beautiful garden and your positive thoughts as flowers in that garden. Cultivate the positive thoughts and weed out

---

Parents' Suggestions:
12 Ways to Take Some Time for Yourself

- "I like to run. I have a group of people I run with. It keeps me sane."
- "When he's absorbed in cartoons, computer games, Game Boy, or Nintendo (and not melting down over his inability to win), then we try to relax."
- "I slowly pursued a hobby of card crafting that has brought me a lot of pleasure."
- "We schedule 'couple's time' and pleasant family outings as often as possible."
- "Little getaways are refreshing. We go to couples' therapy and marriage enrichment weekends."
- "I joined a weight loss group and found supportive women. I stay connected to my husband with our trips to the gym."
- "I found a nonprofit organization in my community that gives money to parents of special needs children for respite every 3 months so I could go exercise or do whatever for a couple of hours a week."
- "My son and I do pottery at a local arts center."
- "Going for a walk with our dog is a great way to get away."
- "I do yoga regularly and sometimes think that I would not stick with it if it weren't for having a bipolar child."
- "The ladies' ministry at church helps me. Going out for coffee with a girlfriend is also great."
- "The 20 minutes of commute time is sort of time to myself."

unhelpful or negative ones and your attitude will bloom. You owe it to yourself to take care of yourself. Care, compassion, and concern are things you owe yourself, as well as the rest of the family.

Reduce Your Stress

When pressure builds up, there are some specific things you can do to reduce your stress level and reestablish your equilibrium. For instance:

Forgive Yourself

Be patient and tolerant with yourself. Forgive yourself for small foibles. Remember, you're going to make mistakes along the way. At times, you will "blow it" with your child. You may lose your temper, be too harsh, or give in when you ought to be firm. We all do. Mistakes are part of the game. The important thing is not that you not make mistakes, but that you recognize them and, when appropriate, apologize for them.

Always remember that you have the right to forgive yourself for being human. One parent said, "None of us are perfect parents . . . we don't come with parent genes, we learn through experiences, talking with others, etc. So, why should we expect that we can parent kids with these challenges without help?" What to do when your human frailty rises to the surface? "Find help and join a support group or get therapy." If you're too embarrassed or confused to seek help at church or another community institution, check out what your local NAMI chapter might offer. Parents frequently comment about how helpful the organization's family-to-family class can be.

Cut Others a Bit of Slack

Whether it's your bipolar child or another family member, it's best to assume that your family's intentions are to do the right thing. While this is not always true, it's always the best assumption with your children, and, if you are going to err, err in this direction. Even when you're wrong, your positive expectations and assumptions will encourage your child to perform according to them. If you're going to have self-fulfilling prophecies, this is the right type to have. In addition, the positive result of cutting others some slack is that there is less stress on you. If you assume that your children want to do the right thing, then when they don't you will find it easier to help them find ways to. This is a variant of the golden rule—think of others as you would have them think of you.

Take Time to Be Alone to Relax and Think

Sometimes we get so busy that we don't have time to regroup and put things in perspective. This takes some time to do and, in today's busy world, doesn't come easily. A regular walk in a quiet spot, an exercise period, or meditation or prayer is what is needed. Whatever your beliefs, this is an important part of a balanced life and a composed mind. If you have a spouse, depend on him or her to be with the kids during this time. If not, get a sitter, or exchange time to watch your friend's kid in return for your watching her kids.

Treasure Times of Relative Happiness

As they say, "take time to smell the roses." Don't expect happiness to last, but do expect it to return. Be sure to notice when your child has a relatively better day and be thankful for it. Praise your child for it. Ponder on it and take pride and pleasure in it. Enjoy other aspects of life that are too easily overlooked: a beautiful sunrise or sunset, a gentle rain, a good grade on your child's homework. Keeping a focus on the positive encourages more positive times to emerge in the future and subtly but surely shapes your child's behavior and the behavior of others around you.

Appreciate Your Own Efforts

You cannot always count on others to appreciate what you do, so you must value it. "I've found the best therapeutic school I can find," said one mother. "I put everything into place that is within my power, and that's all that I can do." Trying to make everything perfect just adds to your stress. Consistently sticking to doing the right thing will remove the largest boulders from your path.

Avoiding Burnout

A parent of a bipolar child can easily get caught up in taking care of everyone else's needs. The rush of events can feel like a car accelerating out of control. Like a car, you can't keep accelerating indefinitely—you *will* either crash or run out of gas. While they consume a lot of energy, your spouse and children should help refuel and recharge you. You shouldn't have to wait until all the kids are grown and out of the house to have a life. You need to take the time to take care of yourself now, so that the whole family can have a promising future to look forward to. Here are some tips for improving your personal life and avoiding burnout.

Get a Hobby

If you don't already have one, get one. If you have had one, get started again and keep it going. It's often better if this is something you do with others, as the commitment will often help you keep on track. Some hobbies are easier than others in that they take less time, are less expensive, or do not demand that you get someone to watch the kids. Regardless, pick something you like, and stick with it. It's not selfish. It's in the interests of your family and everyone else's well-being. Happier parents make happier families.

Diet and Exercise

This is a hard area for all of us. Regularly fitting this into my routine is often tough. For example, my exercise of choice is jogging. It is a lot easier to be consistent if I have committed to a friend or neighbor to show up for a brief run. Similarly, a dieting buddy can provide support and encouragement that can keep you going when your will flags.

Reward Yourself

Go out and do something that you enjoy with someone you trust. See a movie or a concert with a girlfriend, join a book club, or meet for lunch. It will get you out of your daily world and give you a new perspective on your life.

Give Yourself an Allowance

Budget an allowance for yourself. Spend at least as much money on yourself as on your spouse or child. This is hard for some parents. In their minds, kids always come first. You must model self-care and self-caring if you want your child to learn to respect other adults, to be polite, to take others' needs into account, and to respect himself as an adult.

What to Do When Your Personal Life Leaves Something to Be Desired

Parents of children with special needs often feel isolated and put upon. Some say they feel lonely in their own home and have lost touch with their friends because they never go out anymore. Others suddenly notice they're getting sick all the time, or they realize they're always letting their kids or spouse choose the restaurant, leisure activity, vacation site, or dinner menu.

Here are a few tips for solving these personal-life deficits.

Unwind

You may be on the verge of burning out. Too much, too long, basically. It's time to talk with a friend. Sometimes long periods of stress can actually change your brain's neurochemistry, making you prone to depression, excessive alcohol or drug use, or other related problems.

See Your Doctor

Your doctor is in a position to evaluate whether stress has actually caused a depression or other related problem. He can also determine if you have another condition that will make all these tasks and demands even more challenging.

Are You Getting Sufficient Time Alone for Yourself, Really?

You may need to evaluate your R&R (rest and relaxation) opportunities. Are the burdens being shared with your spouse? Can your parents or in-laws help out? Are you keeping up your hobbies?

Revisit the Quality of Your Relationships

Relationships are key to mental health and happiness. It is quite likely that you are not having your needs met in this area. Make sure you review the earlier parts of this chapter, "Taking Care of Yourself."

Back to the Basics

Reevaluate the steps and earlier principles outlined in Chapters 2 and 3.

Is There Life Beyond Bipolar Disorder?

At this point, I hope I have given you the information, encouragement, and basic tools you need to treat childhood bipolar disorder successfully. But you and your child deserve more! You all deserve to have full, satisfying lives, along with opportunities for your child to learn, socialize, pursue interests and experiences, and grow in all aspects of life. That is what I will explore in the next section, along with support for overcoming obstacles and setbacks that can occur along the way.

PART III

Pulling It All Together into Strategies for Specific Situations

WISDOM THAT GETS YOU CENTERED

In Part II, I tried to provide some basic advice on the best approach for treating children with bipolar disorder, along with some proven strategies for working with your treatment providers to improve outcomes for your child, your family, and you. In Part III, I take it one step further and provide additional practical, experienced-based tools and techniques for incorporating these strategies into your daily life, improving your home life, and helping your child maintain the gains she is making through treatment at school, with peers, and in other common situations. In the final chapter, I address mechanisms for dealing with some of the extremely challenging situations that can occasionally result in setbacks and barriers to ongoing progress against the disorder.

The tools and techniques I am about to impart are based on my experience seeing hundreds of families dealing with bipolar disorder in my clinic and research program every year. Informed by brain imaging and cognitive testing, these techniques are built on the proven methods of medication treatment models and the framework of CFF-CBT integrated with interpersonal psychotherapy (i.e., self-psychology), which I discussed in Part

II. I also include ideas and coping strategies from parents who have been in the very same situation. While it is important to understand the psychiatric theory behind these techniques, I know from my clinical experience that theory is not enough—you need a solid tool kit for applying these concepts to the real challenges that come up every day. Therefore, the rest of this book is devoted to sharing these special nuggets of wisdom and insight, along with tips and techniques that families can use to maintain gains at home and away.

EIGHT

Keeping the Peace at Home

"We keep a general order to our home, but not rigid. For example, clutter is kept to a minimum. The house is clean enough. We don't use a lot of bright lights or loud music. We play soft music, light candles. Kids are welcome to come over to the house to play—two at a time max. We eat dinner together at least four times a week."

Wouldn't it be great if there was some way to make life with a bipolar child go well all the time? We'd all like more days when life is in balance, the morning and evening routine go easily, everyone gets along and homework gets done, you get a lot of support from your spouse and other family members, and the teacher doesn't call with a new problem to address. But, as you well know by now, it rarely goes that way. My advice to you is to let go of that expectation. Life means change—with or without a bipolar child—so do yourself a favor and accept the inevitable ups and downs.

More often than not, the day starts with a fight about getting up and getting off to school. Your child dawdles, there's fussing and yelling, the other children get caught up in finding your bipolar child's shoes, and finally everyone races for the car. You get a call from school saying your child has had an outburst and needs to be picked up. You run to the doctor's office to get a prescription for some new medications. When you get home, the TV goes on and you can't get your child to focus on homework. The battle continues through dinner and beyond, until bedtime, when everyone collapses in exhaustion just to do the whole thing again the next day.

If perfect days are out of reach, what can you expect? With a little effort, flexibility, and a sense of humor, you can have a moderately successful household routine that works reasonably well for you and other family members. As Benjamin Franklin put it, "everything in moderation"; and that holds true for establishing order and discipline at home.

How to Establish a Balanced Routine

"Each day is an uncertainty as to whether the rollercoaster will be going up, down, or both. Will my son be in the mood to get up out of bed and go to school? Will he react aggressively to a comment that others perceive as normal? Will there be a meltdown over the tiniest thing? Will he call us names or embarrass us in public?"

I know I've addressed this in several places already, but I can't emphasize enough how important a consistent and balanced routine is to your child's mood stability (and your sanity). See Chapter 6 for suggestions for establishing daily routines, and keep in mind that there are five important aspects of your child's daily routine that need attending to: getting up, eating breakfast, going to school, doing homework, and bedtime. If you can establish a reasonable amount of structure for your child around these five daily activities, you will have achieved a lot.

Of these daily touch points, bedtime may be the most important, and some suggestions for climbing this mountain without constantly sliding backward are in Chapter 6. Sleep is important for you, too, allowing you to refill your psychic reservoir so you have more to offer your child. I often get long e-mails from sleep-deprived parents pouring their hearts out about how exhausting it is to deal with their bipolar child into the small hours of the morning, how they never have any personal adult time in the evening, and so on. That is why I urge parents to get their child's sleep routine under control for everyone's sake.

Beyond a good sleep routine, your family schedule should include at least one meal a day together. Homework can be scheduled before or after dinner, along with showers or baths. The timetable should be neither so strict that it frustrates both you and your child nor so loose that chaos reins. The goal is to strike a balance that works for all of you. If homework is a major stumbling block, you should get a note from your doctor asking the school to reduce the amount of homework or tailor it to your child's capacity, unless your child is already in a therapeutic school.

Guiding Principles for Keeping Peace at Home

A central principle for having a reasonable if not peaceful home life is keeping things in perspective. Decide what really matters to you and let everything else go. Use your journal to write a list of essentials and nonessentials that you can refer to when you feel yourself floundering in wave after wave of responsibilities. If we're honest with ourselves, we realize that most of our problems are small and insignificant, and few things are of life-and-death importance. Keeping a firm grip on this principle will serve you well when real crises erupt. Here are some other helpful suggestions to keep in mind. You've heard some of these before in slightly different words, but I think they bear repeating because I want you to remember that when solutions to problems at home and elsewhere seem to elude you, you can always return to the well of basic principles for novel ideas.

Establish Parental Control

Many parents of bipolar children feel controlled by their child's angry and irritable moods and bossiness, which is bad for both parent and child. Parents must assert their natural role and set the kinds of limits that make children feel more secure. This is not one of the small things that can be let go of! These children generally know right from wrong and that their efforts to "get their way" are out of line. Believe it or not, they want you to step in and help them establish boundaries. You don't owe them an explanation or justification when they are being bossy, demanding, or controlling or pushing you. Tell them what is expected of them and keep it at that. Don't let them negotiate over every little thing. They are smart enough to yield if you remain firm. So why let the currency be lost by yielding to every request? Anchor yourself. Set expectations. Keep some things normal.

Set Realistic Expectations

Keep your expectations realistic and don't stress out about little things. Don't go overboard with ambitious plans. Remember, you have plenty of battles to fight, and maybe keeping the house perfectly clean is asking a bit too much at this point. Getting your child to school on time, helping him get homework done, and managing and keeping your own job are all significant achievements in and of themselves.

Pick Your Battles

You can't win every battle, so don't even try. Focus instead on winning the war: keeping your child and your home functioning reasonably well without burning yourself out on trivial things that won't matter in the long run. In making the system work for your child with bipolar disorder, you have lots of areas to tackle, and your personal energy is needed in many places. Are household routines and chores really an important issue right now? *The* most important issue? Or is reconnecting as a family and just doing something fun together likely to refuel you for the coming week more than the cleanest and neatest house could possibly do? If you really want the neatest house, plan on involving kids in helping you so that you can achieve your goals. If they want a reward for helping out, why not give them one?

Compromise

If your spouse and other adult family members aren't cooperating, it might make sense to compromise and set different goals that others can support. It's hard to pull this off if the other adults in the home aren't pulling with you. Remember, the only one you can control is yourself. But you can tap your problem-solving skills with the adults in your life just as you do with your bipolar child. Consult your list of essentials and nonessentials to see where you might be willing to yield a bit as a start.

Communicate Clearly

It is important that house rules, tasks, and assignments be written down and posted where others can see them so there's no second-guessing. You might find a whiteboard with dry-erase markers helpful, perhaps posted close to the refrigerator or by the phone.

Reduce Reactivity

There are times your child will be completely defiant and drive you into the worst possible rage; you are likely to become explosive yourself. In fact, parents often develop their own version of bipolar-type reactivity as a defense against their child's difficult attacks. You need to check this in yourself, but it does happen now and again. It is OK for your child to hear that you are upset with her behavior—it's a form of feedback. Forgive yourself for blowing off a little steam. After it's over, let go of it and move on. One parent had a counselor who told her, "It's OK not to like your child's illness because you love your child, and if you always remember you love your child, the rest is just fluff, and the fluff always goes away." But remember that your feelings of anger and dislike, love and tenderness are like a rollercoaster ride that is natural for most mothers and fathers. If you don't have these ups and downs, you are either a monk in the Himalayas or a person without normal human emotional capacity! You can get yourself back to a state of love and compassion by a thought process such as: "My child is hurting. I will not ridicule or negate my child. I will make it better by loving him. Loving does not always mean saying yes or yielding." The more you show compassion, the more addictive it gets to be that way! This does *not* mean being a "softie" who is manipulated by your child or becoming ineffective. It means bringing a sense of compassion that helps you do all you need to do with love and passion and strengthens your will to grin and bear it until you reach the stage when you can look back on the struggles and chuckle smugly at how far you've come.

Do Things in Small Bits

Take on challenges a little bit at a time, rather than biting off more than you, your child, and your family can chew. Give your child information in small pieces if she is likely to react excitably. This strategy can be invaluable when handling special occasions that can be particularly stimulating, such as birthdays and holidays; one parent said, "Christmas is done in small bites: one present before we leave, then at Grandma's, then at the next stop, to help diffuse the building up of anticipation that is hard for them." Some parents allow their child to retreat to his bedroom during large family gatherings to avoid chaos. Act as a buffer or moderator or adapt the situation to keep the intensity down.

Allow Extra Time

Expect things to take more time, so schedule fewer in a day and be ready for a change in plans. Try not to rush around—just go with the flow and keep the plan flexible. One parent said, "If we need to spend extra time on the road, we will. If we need to return home early, we will. Whatever happens, we'll adjust. That's the attitude you need to go into it with." You are more of a superwoman (or superman) if you slow down and pace yourself, rather than trying to do it all.

Keep a Sense of Humor

Keep your sense of humor and don't get too lost in a bad moment. Being lighthearted and mellow helps reduce tension and keeps things in perspective. "Once, in the middle of a rage," reports one mother, "my son turned a garden hose on me, full in the face. What could I do? I burst into laughter. That's not always the best approach, but it has saved my sanity a number of times." Another adds, "Who else endures such bizarre and extreme behaviors from their children? Who else has had to be as creative as I have in my parenting? Some days, I just chuckle to myself and think, 'I can't wait to tell the girls in my online support group what he just did/said/etc.'"

Ask a Friend

There's lots of wisdom out there about how to manage a household, and no one is born knowing how to do it. A lot can be learned through trial and error and feedback from friends. See if you can get some advice from someone who has been there. You can get a great deal of solace from having that heart-to-heart conversation. It might be helpful to touch base with another parent who has a bipolar child, join a support group, or get on a bulletin board to commiserate or get ideas on a more regular basis.

Empathize and Collaborate

Imagine yourself in your child's shoes (or out of them) and approach problems in a sympathetic, collaborative manner. One parent said, "I try to remember that it's not my child saying mean things and acting crazy, but the disease."

Schedule One-on-One Time

Try to schedule a regular time with your child—just his time, no one else's—when you pursue an activity that your child likes and can help choose and that you can enjoy together. You might feel guilty about doing this, as your bipolar child probably already takes the lion's share of attention in your family. We all want to give our children equal attention, but, in this situation, you should recognize that realistically the bipolar child must get the larger share of the pie.

Maid to Order

Just a bit of extra help, even once a month, may make a great deal of difference to your peace of mind if this issue continues to weigh on you. This is especially valuable if you and your partner are constantly arguing about your share of work.

How Can You Lighten Your Load at Home?

Parents of bipolar children frequently feel like they are carrying the weight of the world on their shoulders, and sometimes one spouse (often the mother) carries the majority of the load. If you are the most "tuned in" to your child's moods and have the most experience managing your child's behavior, you may feel like it's all up to you to keep things together at home.

But sharing the load with other members of the family is essential, even if it's just getting them to keep things tidy or set the table or make meals a couple of times a week. Your bipolar child should also have responsibilities, even if they are somewhat simplified, so that she can contribute to the family's functioning whenever possible.

Your spouse, other relatives, or even a capable babysitter can take on some of the caregiving burden so you can find time to recharge and refresh, as described in Chapter 7.

Get Everyone Helping around the House

You and your spouse, as well as your children, must share in the various responsibilities of running the household. If it is all on your back, and you find yourself always the one picking up the slack, it's time to evaluate and adjust roles and patterns.

While it may seem like too much trouble to expect a young child, even a 3-year-old, to help, if you don't start now, it will get harder (but not impossible) later. Regardless of what you have done in the past, let's set a new rule: everyone in the family who can speak and understand simple requests is a part of your team to handle household chores. This is not a Holiday Inn, and you are not a maid or bellboy. Simple tasks, such as picking up, hanging up one's coat, putting books and schoolwork away, and caring for personal items is required for every family member. This includes your spouse, your child with bipolar disorder, and your other kids.

It might be useful to create some household routines that involve all the family's members. For example, you can make picking up toys before bedtime a game and have a little race or fun contest to put the toys away as quickly as possible. Other ideas include having your children make their beds before leaving for school or assigning five or six different routine household chores (e.g., vacuuming, emptying trash, sweeping the floors, cleaning the bathrooms, etc.), for which children get to rotate jobs on a regular basis. An example is a simple strategy for daily dishes: each child picks a day of the week to wash the dishes.

Should the Bipolar Child Be Asked to Do Chores?

Unequivocally, yes. It's an opportunity for him to take a leadership role, which can be very motivating and reinforce positive behavior. Helping your bipolar child assume responsibility is doubly important if there is more than one child in the family; it will stoke anger and jealousy if the bipolar child always seems to get off easy. What this means is that he or she will still have to bear reasonably similar responsibilities to your other children, although at times you will have to offer extra support or even assist him.

You may think I am talking out of both sides of my mouth, and I am, but for good reason. There are times bipolar kids are fragile and go through phases of instability. Knowing when not to push is very important. Wear the hat of compassion and let go in tough times. In addition, there are just some bad days apart from ill phases. During these times, don't go toe-to-toe to make a point. *Let go* once in a while. This is not a case of inconsistency, but realistically accommodating an illness-related disability! I know I've said it before, but it bears repeating: stick to rules, but be ready to go with the flow.

Each family is different, so you'll have to ask yourself what's really important for you. What gets most under your skin? Maybe it's the empty orange juice container left in the fridge or the mud tracked into the kitchen or things left around that you feel like you have to pick up? The issue might not be housekeeping-related at all, but the driving around you must do or shopping or paying bills. How might these tasks be divvied up or your burdens lessened? How about setting some limits or rules, like no more than one or two extracurricular activities per week? Or state that you'll drive once a week to soccer practice, also taking your child's friends to it, but that for the other two times per week, other parents or your spouse will have to step in? If your child is old enough, it might be possible for him or her to arrange her own ride. Don't feel guilty about setting limits. As much as possible, your child needs a rested, patient, unharried parent.

Encourage Teamwork and Fair Play

Having and taking time for yourself also teaches important principles to your child with bipolar disorder and to other family members in that it models the idea that basic respect for others and teamwork are necessary parts of life. Don't avoid defending your own needs because that will inadvertently teach your children that it's OK to walk on you. It's not. Making sure that your own needs are met, particularly when it means that others must give a little, teaches citizenship and fair play.

Parents sometimes make the mistake of having the entire family revolve around meeting the children's needs. While children do, indeed, have many needs and are somewhat more dependent on adults than adults are on children, it is still a two-way street. So, for the long-term benefit to your children's character, you can and should insist that your children consider your needs, including the need for your own activities and time alone and their assistance in making that possible. Of course, the same rule must apply to other family members; you can and should expect your child with bipolar disorder and siblings to respect each other's rights and needs.

Don't Forget to Have Fun

All work and no play makes everyone cranky! If families were meant only to clothe, feed, and house kids, an orphanage or a youth hostel would be a much cheaper option. Remember, your home should be a safe haven, a sanctuary where adults and children can bond and feel understood and accepted by each other (at least sometimes!), where family members can relax, have fun, and be spontaneous. So, in all of the efforts you expend on assisting your bipolar child, relax and have fun together. Refer to the guiding principles earlier in this chapter: many of them are based on realism, compassion, and balance. When we apply these at home, they can make living there a lot happier.

There are many ways to increase the fun factor in your home. Just taking time to dine together and talk at the table can put a new perspective on things. Take monthly outings together and special birthday trips. As long as household chores and homework were done, one family I know would plan outings that were enjoyable and fun for all of them on a weekly basis—skating, movies, pizza, zoo, baseball game, museum. Make opportunities for downtime, such as "PJ days" and "cuddle-up time" to recharge yourselves emotionally. Let us get this straight. These "least scheduled family days" are purposeful; they don't automatically happen unless you give them the space to. Create an island of healthy life that you and your child can retreat to when needed.

Keeping Your Marriage Healthy

Having a bipolar child takes a toll on many marriages. When there is denial about the diagnosis or even the existence of the disorder in children, it can sometimes be viewed in terms of a parenting or "discipline" failure. Often, this is accompanied by a battle in which one partner, frequently the father, refuses to allow the child to be medicated. It is not uncommon to see a wife and husband heatedly disagree about this issue.

Sometimes one parent (usually the father) assumes that, because the bipolar child behaves better for him than for the other parent, the other parent is just not a good disciplinarian or is too much of a pushover. This notion is almost always incorrect and fails to account for the different dynamics of the child's relationship with his mother and father. A fearful child may *temporarily* respond to a father's gruff command or foreboding physical presence, but if that same father had to do all of the parenting, day in and day out, the novelty would wear off, and the child would eventually show just as many behavioral difficulties and noncompliance as with the parent he spends more time with (even in today's society, this is still usually the mother). When one parent "blows in" and barks a command to the child, all the while subtly blaming the other parent for not being more like him, strong negative forces begin to operate on the marital relationship. One parent had her husband take a week of vacation to be in the house with their child while she went elsewhere. After day two, he "got it."

Another common problem is when a triangle develops in which the child and one parent gang up against the other parent—either mom and child versus dad or dad and child versus mom—often made worse if there has already been a divorce. Because of the potential for hypersexuality, this dynamic can become intensified with bipolar children where the child can get flirtatious with the parent of the opposite sex (this is not necessarily sexualized beyond flirtation). All of these issues can drive a wedge between partners and wreck a marriage. If you and your spouse are wrangling over these situations, it may be worth seeking marriage counseling.

Finally, given the genetic source of bipolar disorder, there can be a lot of finger-pointing in which one spouse can be blamed for "passing it on" (and sometimes a sense of guilt convinces the parent he is culpable). Conflict over how to treat or raise the bipolar child, assigning of blame, and emotional manipulation by the child can wreak havoc over the long term in a marriage, generating resentment, arguments, and increasing emotional distance. Don't let this fester; instead, make it an issue for discussion and problem solving early on, rather than after it has clogged up your communication channels.

First Aid for Your Marriage

Focus on the Positive

Celebrate the good times, ignore the negative, and make special times to be together—that's my personal rule of thumb for maintaining a happy marriage when you have a bipolar child in the house, or even if you don't. Take the time to empathize with your partner and see it from his or her point of view. Remember how you used to look adoringly into each other's eyes as newlyweds? Those passionate moments produce positive energy that keeps the emotional bank account full. When the account is empty, it is hard to get the chariot of love going steady! We all need our egos to be fed, have others empathize with us, and feel nurtured. One very good way to do this is to give positive feedback and compliment the things your spouse does right. One mother said she used to make a point of complimenting her husband on something he did well during the day with regard to their child. You might say something like, "I loved that you called in the morning to check on Tom"; "I hope you have had some rest"; "Can I get this for you?"; "How about I give you a back rub?"; or "I want you to hold me because I love you." There are times when you will need to provide constructive criticism, for instance, reminding your spouse to stay compassionate with your child. But it is still best to let most things go and not bring up hurts and failures from the past. Keep moving forward. Get up and start again each time you fall down and skin your knee. If it is impossible to do this on your own, seek help from a therapist or other counselor who can put a little perspective on the situation.

Share the Challenges

If you are reading this book, chances are you are on the front lines, involved in more of the daily battles than your spouse. You may feel that you need to shield your spouse from the reality of caring for your child, particularly if he tends to be critical of your parenting skills. If you do this, your spouse may not have a realistic idea of what's possible or fully appreciate the challenges you face. Take a few days or up to a week off so he or she can better understand what you're up against.

Divide and Conquer

A good marriage should be approximately 50–50, but in the short run, it may be 70–30 or even 20–80. If one parent has an illness or a particularly bad time at work, the other may carry more of the burden. If you are bearing more of the burden, this has to be acknowledged, and there has to be trust and mutual support that it will balance out over time. But if marriage partners are busy counting who did what and who owes whom how much, something is awry. Trust and genuine sharing of responsibilities cannot be handled like legal contracts, and if a marriage is headed in that direction, it is time to get some counseling.

Give and Get Appreciation

You need and deserve thanks and appreciation for all you do, but don't expect your spouse to read your mind. So don't fall into the common trap of thinking, "If she *really* cared, then she would know that. . . ." Tell her what she need. Communicating your needs, including your needs for appreciation, is your responsibility. It is the other partner's responsibility to provide it. But mind reading was not in the marriage vows. Nonetheless, because misunderstandings can so frequently arise when a family is under stress, it might be a good rule of thumb to actively look for ways to show each other your appreciation.

Spend Time as a Couple

For a marriage to survive the stress of having a child with bipolar disorder, you'll need time to get away together by yourselves. A weekly outing or date or even just a regular walk together is critical to keeping this relationship intact. And you must talk about things other than your child. What interests did you share when you got married? What are your interests and hobbies? What happened in your spouse's day that made him happy? Or sad? What went well? What was the hardest thing about her day? This needs to be shared in a two-way fashion. It's good for you to ask these questions and listen, but don't forget to ask for and expect the same in return.

If You Have to Go It Alone

Sometimes the stress of raising a bipolar child will be too much for a couple and they will split up, leaving one spouse to go it alone. It is even more important that single parents offload some of the household burdens onto other family members or paid help and find assistance caring for the bipolar child. Otherwise, they risk complete burnout. For single parents, girlfriends, grandparents, teachers, neighbors, church friends, friends at work, babysitters (if you can afford them), aunts, and uncles are possible sources of support. While it can be a relief to end an unhappy relationship with an uncooperative or negative spouse, the logistical challenges of doing it all alone can be overwhelming. Cut it down to bite-size pieces and count on expanding your list of resources.

Finding a Babysitter or Other Respite

You're probably thinking, "Time to get away—are you kidding? Who would stay with my child?" Finding a babysitter or leaving a sibling in charge may seem like the impossible dream, especially if your child is going through a particularly turbulent phase. "*Who would be responsible for the 13 pills in the morning and 12 pills at night? Who could calm my child when he gets a panic attack full of anxiety about someone breaking in to hurt him? Who would take care of my child when he is vomiting from a bad mix of meds or comfort him when his hand tremors just won't stop?"* You may have the same kinds of questions as this mother.

There's no question that not everyone is qualified for or capable of taking care of a bipolar child. A sibling may be too young or close to the bipolar child to take charge effectively. A mature teenager or college student could be appropriate, but you should be prepared to invest some time coaching, training, and monitoring her to ensure that she can handle the medication, behavioral strategies, and simple safety issues connected with your child's care. See the box for some tips on how to prepare others to care for your child.

It may take a lot of work to find the right person, but once you do, you'll want to use his or her assistance whenever possible. One family I know of found a nanny to go on vacations with them and actually traveled separately to give themselves a little break:

> *"We drive the 15 hours in the car and she flies out with our son to join us a day or two later. Her sole responsibility is keeping him entertained and calm and safe. With three adults to one bipolar kid, we*

What to Look for in a Babysitter

- High-energy young males are good for boys, as they never get exhausted, love to play, and weave in work in between! They may take your child to baseball games too.
- Affectionate young women are good for girls.
- Knowing that your babysitter works in a credible aftercare facility or local day care gives you assurance that she is checked to be safe with respect to child care.
- Word of mouth is the best and safest way to get babysitters.
- Check at the local university or reputable high school.
- Friends of nieces and nephews are good.
- Bringing in an au pair from a reputable agency can be a good way to get constant support for little or no cost.
- Finally, there are no guarantees! Your astute judgment and luck play a major role.

have him outmanned. Then, when it's time to come home, we drop them off at the airport and meet them back home the next day. Saved our lives!"

Money can also be an issue, as one spouse often leaves work to care for the bipolar child, giving the family only one income. In this case, asking a patient and understanding relative, trading with another parent whose child has similar problems, or contacting respite services from your local agencies may be a more affordable, realistic alternative.

Improving Sibling Relationships

All kids fight and pick on each other, but this can take on greater intensity in a family that includes a bipolar child. The bipolar child's extreme sensitivity and volatility can produce incredible friction in the family that can turn a simple car trip into a real nightmare.

It takes good management skills on your part to maintain relative peace. Siblings should be educated about bipolar disorder and expected to behave with compassion and understanding. Teasing and taunting of the bipolar child should be strictly prohibited, although, obviously, this needs to be a two-way street. Often, the bipolar child is jealous of the "normal" siblings and might tease and taunt them, find their weaknesses, and target them for put-downs. Bipolar children may see their parents as not loving them as much as their siblings and may resent any attention paid to siblings. Any perceived threat to the parental relationship may trigger a reaction from the bipolar child.

I advise you to separate the bipolar child from her siblings to provide each with his or her own space. Once you establish separate spheres of activity, such as separate play dates or extracurricular activities, tension can be reduced and they may tolerate one another better.

Be patient, repeat yourself a lot, give consistent praise and rewards for getting along, and dish out regular consequences without getting too upset when things get contentious. If the conflict becomes relentless or your bipolar child becomes violent or extremely depressed or threatens a sibling's or his own safety, you might have to consider hospitalization or even removing him from the home for residential placement. See the next section for more help dealing with these kinds of extreme challenges.

Tips for Helping Siblings Cope

I know you are thinking about how to protect your other children when they are suffering from the attacks and slights of the bipolar child. What I normally do is to have parents watch me as I explain how to handle this situation. I expect parents to perpetuate the teachings at home. Here's what I suggest:

- First, empathize with the siblings from time to time. Understand how hard it is to be a child living with another angry, irritable child.
- Listen to them till they are completely done venting to you. Stop questioning and correcting. Pause. Empathize some more.
- Then explain how especially hard it is for the bipolar child to face the symptoms, feel rejected, and fail at lot of things and how hard it is to make it at school and get along.
- Teach the siblings a few tricks to respond in the midst of dealing with their bipolar sibling. Get them to say "Whatever"; "So?"; "Leave me alone"; "Enough is enough"; "I don't like it"; "Please stop it," and so on.
- Get them to pepper their conversations with empathy or loving sentences. Teach them that, when in doubt, they can try active listening—"You must be feeling kind of bad right now" or "I'd feel that way too" or "This must be really hard for you"—when the bipolar is saying or doing something that makes it clear he's in distress.
- Teach your other children actively to support the ill child in the family. Look at it like volunteering to help serve in a soup kitchen or read magazines to geriatric patients. The difference is they are volunteering at home to a very sick sibling. Make it a conscious decision and an adventure, a proactive "Giving Act."
- Help the siblings understand that it is not just you, but all of you as a team, that must pitch in to engage, influence, and help the bipolar child. Hug them as you teach them! Influence them to be their best selves.

Extreme Challenges

Sometimes, despite your best efforts, your child and you will go through very difficult times. In some cases, the situation may become so challenging as to constitute a crisis that you may not know how to handle. Severe mood swings, continuing problems at school, substance abuse, risky behavior, sexual acting out, and suicide attempts fall into this category. So does any situation in which the child is a danger to herself or others. I discuss school problems in Chapter 9 and self-harm in Chapter 5. The following are some extreme behavior problems you might encounter and some ideas for handling them. In general, be prepared for the possibility that your child will be "precocious" in engaging in some of these behaviors as a result of the nature of bipolar disorder.

Family Conflict and Violence

"Our son was dangerous to live with for about a year, and there were times when I feared that he would kill himself, if not me. He still refuses to believe that he could have killed me the time that he grabbed me around my throat."

As we have discussed throughout this book, there can be times when life can feel like a war zone for everyone in the family, with small conflicts escalating into full-blown violence on a regular basis. Parents often take the brunt of this behavior and are frequently its target because Mom and Dad are close to the child, who feels entitled when it comes to dealing with parents. Parents talk about having to restrain their child for an hour or more until such rages pass. As your child grows older and larger, you may no longer feel you have the strength to do this, and you may have to admit to yourself that you have limited control over your child's illness and the eventual outcome. Recognize when it's time to get help from your doctor, the mental health system, or even the police if the situation spirals out of control. Involving the police usually is not an option unless the child is so violent that it is like having a tiger in the home, and you need help transporting him to a hospital. If the child is raging like a wild animal for several hours, tearing the home apart, or may harm or even kill someone, you ought to consider calling for help to take him to the hospital. Using police sounds drastic but is not unreasonable if no one can help you take him via ambulance.

Even if there is no immediate physical threat, a high level of family conflict can have other negative effects on family members. The toll may show up in a number of ways, including anxiety, depression, and bipolar-type reactive behavior in other family members. Frequent breaks for other children may be needed; sending them to a neighbor's house or to visit grandparents is one way to break the tension. Providing a safe outlet for other family members, who may feel high levels of guilt, responsibility, or shame, is critically important. Siblings, parents, and other members of the household need a place where they can speak honestly with a third party about how they feel about living with the bipolar child and deal with their fears, anxiety, and exhaustion from having to cope with the bipolar child's extreme behavior. This can be informal—through a church, support group, or school counselor—or formal, through therapy. Almost all insurance companies will pay for collateral visits, where other family members can be seen as a means of assisting the primary patient. In addition, if you or your other children are suffering from depression, post-traumatic stress disorder, or another related condition, you may be eligible for coverage as well. Temporary out-of-home placement or hospitalization may be necessary for youngsters who cannot be safely maintained in their own home.

Risky Behavior

Risky behavior is a common symptom of bipolar disorder, and children may engage in it as early as 6–7 years of age. This behavior, as well as some parents' methods of coping with it, can set off alarms among well-meaning but misinformed bystanders and even helping professionals. One parent described how her daughter would launch herself over the back of the front seat and open the passenger door while they were driving on the highway. Because the car's child locks didn't work on the front door, her husband had to rig a lock and chain on the door. Other parents talk about sleeping outside their child's door to keep her from slipping out at night or even attempting to lock the child in.

While it may be tempting to take such extreme measures to protect your child from himself, don't go overboard! You could be placing your child at even greater risk and setting yourself up for potential legal problems. First, try to get the behavior under control with medication and therapy. If all else fails, the child may need to be hospitalized for a period of time or placed in a residential treatment program until this behavior abates.

Hypersexuality

As we discussed in Chapter 2, some sexual acting out can be mistaken for symptoms of abuse and lead to false accusations and family strife, which can be devastating. Parents report behaviors such as grabbing at their breasts, saying "I love you" to the parent of the opposite sex over and over in public places, and even using highly sexually charged language at a very young age. As children age, use of "dirty words" and provocative behavior can lead to real problems outside the home. Preteens might dress provocatively and have trouble with the school dress code. They might engage in underage sexual behavior and suffer a variety of consequences.

It is important to address this subject when you coach and teach your child, even though it might make you feel uncomfortable or embarrassed. Hopefully, medication and therapy will help tone down the more extreme forms hypersexuality can take. Take the time to correct this behavior early on and teach your child to cope with disappointments, need for approval, and unhealthy ways of seeking attention. Establish the boundaries for acceptable and unacceptable behavior very early to provide a stable set of values that will help carry your child through these mood-based behaviors.

Self-Medicating through Substance Abuse

This is an issue that crops up mainly in teenagers as they try to "self-medicate" to deal with their difficult feelings and relationships. Marijuana is often the drug of choice for bipolar teens. Illegal drug use is a problem in and of itself, as it can interfere with the child's carefully managed medication regimen and destabilize mood, but it also puts the child into contact with the "wrong crowd," promoting an antiauthoritarian attitude, school avoidance, and a spiraling cascade of negative events.

In this case, an ounce of prevention is worth a pound of cure. Teaching your child about the risks associated with substance abuse and his particular susceptibility to drug use can help you head off this problem. Keeping a careful watch on peer relationships and helping your child develop healthy methods of coping with his frustrations is critical.

Looking ahead, if your child's substance abuse continues throughout adolescence, you may be able to buy yourself some parental supervision time. I often work with parents to extend guardianship beyond 18 years for just this reason. If that strategy fails and the substance use and negative peer influences continue to grow, it may be necessary to move your child to a different environment, such as a residential treatment center, where there is strong supervision and control. Remember, once she reaches age 21, you will no longer have that option, so early intervention is a much better option!

Suicidality and Suicide Attempts

Suicide is among every parent's greatest fears, and, unfortunately, bipolar children may threaten to harm or kill themselves even at a very young age. Studies indicate a significantly higher rate of suicide attempts and completions among bipolar teens than among those with simple depression or no mental illness.

Bipolar disorder is in and of itself a suicide risk factor, along with the presence of comorbid conditions such as depression, conduct disorders, anxiety, substance abuse, psychosis, and borderline personality disorder and a history of suicidal thoughts or attempts. It is also more common among males over the age of 14. In addition, the risk increases when the child experiences problems in the following areas:

- **Psychological, social, or academic problems** (school failure; social ostracism or isolation; conflict with teacher, family, and peers; poor impulse control and problem-solving capabilities)
- **Family trauma** (physical/sexual abuse or neglect, death or divorce in the family, family history of mood disorders or suicide, stressful school or community environment and media exposure)
- **Physical vulnerability** (chronic illness, substance abuse, hopeless attitude, and availability of guns, pills, and other methods of self-injury).

Children and teenagers are at greatest risk for suicide during a depressive or mixed episode, while transitioning between mood states, or at times of crisis (real or imagined).

What Are the Signs to Watch for?

With suicide as a frame of reference, we see a wide variation in the way children indicate suicidal intentions. One thing that seems to be clear to me is that morbidity and depth of distress are definitely higher in the bipolar child who expresses suicidal ideation or gestures. One parent I know commented how it broke her heart hearing her child say he wanted to kill himself at age 6. Some children make statements like "I wish I am dead"; "I wish you did not have to put up with me if I am dead"; and "I want to be with Nana in heaven." Some actually take drug overdoses, recklessly use recreational drugs, or use a knife on themselves and/or others in a frenzied mood. They draw melodramatic pictures of the ways they want to die. Some slit their wrists or scratch their arms to the point of bleeding to express their rage. (Note that self-injury is not always a sign of suicidality, as discussed below, although some self-injurers do harbor suicidal thoughts.)

How Should You React?

I take any sign that a child is thinking about injuring or killing himself seriously and work to find a solution on a case-by-case basis. This is a delicate area, but most doctors will tell you that any suicidal thoughts, talk of suicide, or suicide attempts should be taken seriously and help sought immediately. It is not something I like to write, but kids also sometimes say this at the drop of a hat to provoke you. Whether said in anger and frustration or with serious intent, a reference to suicide provides important information that your child is hurting. Notice it, listen to it, discuss it, address it, and get help.

Some parents worry about whether to talk to their children about suicide. Will doing so put the idea in their heads? Research indicates that talking about suicide does *not* increase the chance that a child will think about or act on it. Believe me, children hear about the idea from news reports, movies, and peers, so this is your chance to set the record straight and share your values. Share your feelings about suicide even if you only suspect your child may be having suicidal thoughts. Tell her how precious life is. Teach your child that suicide is never an answer to what is troubling her and that a single impulsive act can have a permanent effect (with children and even adolescents, the permanency of death will be hard to grasp). Whether your child brings the subject up or you start the conversation because you think he might be having suicidal thoughts, it is important that your child know you are there for him and want to help and protect him. Tell him you care and that you take him seriously. Validate his feelings. Be strong, no matter how hard it is. Train yourself to listen to his feelings even if you don't want to.

If your child is thinking about suicide or has made an attempt, here's what you should do:

- Take any threats seriously—never dismiss suicidal talk or self-harm as attention-seeking behavior.
- Don't panic or become angry or judgmental.

- Listen to your child and use it as an opportunity to find out how she is feeling.
- Remove available methods, including medications, to prevent "accidents."
- Supervise your child closely (24-7) until the crisis has passed.
- Seek hospitalization if your child is psychotic, agitated, talks about or tries to commit suicide, or has tried in the past and won't promise not to try again.
- Outpatient management will depend on how much supervision is needed and your ability to maintain it.
- With a teen, you should make a "no-suicide contract" in which he agrees to talk to the doctor, his parents, or a hotline if he begins to contemplate suicide again; this is not foolproof, but at least you engaged him.
- One of the most dangerous culprits for teens is a toxic peer influence that can include drugs, morbid music, risky behavior, and other dangers. Encouraging alternative friendships or arranging a school away from this type of peer is a welcome solution.
- Treatment should include medication to stabilize mood, along with therapy and tools specifically designed to address suicidal thoughts, such as compassionate listening, minimizing the tendency to overdramatize crises without patronizing, giving hope, and providing concrete strategies for coping and skills that can be practiced to overcome distress.

What about Self-Injury?

"My daughter used to be very depressed and was self-mutilating. I used to wake up in the morning and think if this is the day that I will lose my daughter."

Cutting and self-mutilation are seen quite often in bipolar children and can be associated with suicidal behavior but may be separate. Whether your child's cutting is related to suicide or not, it needs to be addressed with your doctor. When I hear that a child is cutting herself and there is no history of abuse, I try to address the anger and inner turmoil that is often associated with bipolar illness. Have your physician evaluate your child if this behavior continues or shows any sign of escalating.

These behaviors lead some to think that these children or teens have borderline personality disorder (or are "borderlines to be"), but they often do not have the abuse history associated with teens who are borderline.

Taking a Break from the Routine

"I went on as many field trips with her and her class as I could, and for the most part had a great time! She was popular at summer camp—they actually had a week in her honor when we moved! We went to most of her sporting events, and she did well, although sometimes she could be a bit extreme. She would call the whole team on her own initiative if there was some doubt if enough would show up for a game. Vacations were usually OK, although once I had to borrow my sister's babysitter to fly with us when I was worried that I'd need help if things were to get out of control."

As we discussed earlier, it is possible to establish a workable routine that can be sustained for long periods of time. However, you, your child, and the rest of your family shouldn't be limited to a dull daily routine because of this disorder. That would not only be boring, but it would also be unfair to everyone involved!

Bipolar children and their families deserve to have a full, well-rounded life, with the same opportunities as anyone else to go out and have a good time, take trips and vacations, and celebrate holidays and special occasions. Your child has the same right and need as any other child to go on field trips or to summer camp or to pursue a sport or hobby. Given the stress factor and potential for embarrassment in public (not to mention interfering relatives) that can accompany these events, it might be tempting to avoid them or even cut them out of your lives completely, but don't do it! As I said earlier, all work and no play makes everyone cranky. You and your child need these breaks from the routine to bond, recharge emotionally, and explore who you are as individuals and as a family.

Let me make one other point: if you limit yourself to the school–work–home shuffle, you will go buggy after a while! Planning an occasional getaway with your spouse or going on a retreat with girlfriends can give you a fresh perspective and restore your spirit. Even in your job, there might be times when you need or want to travel to a conference or to see a customer that make it absolutely necessary to change the usual program.

You have to be ready to make accommodations to make these things possible, for the sake of your career as well as your sanity.

So how do you survive and maybe even enjoy these breaks from the routine? How can everyone have a better experience when on car trips or family vacations, at holiday gatherings, or just out shopping? Are school outings, extracurricular activities, sports, and camps out of the question, or are there ways to make sure your bipolar child can get and stay involved?

Here, again, you must be ready to wear your manager's hat and make a realistic yet flexible plan for out-of-the ordinary situations. As wonderful as it would be to let things just happen, nine times out of ten, that approach will lead to disappointment and frustration. So you need to be proactive and try to follow several basic rules:

- *Manage medications:* Be sure your child is appropriately medicated and use rescue medication if needed. For instance, I knew of one bipolar child who went on a 13-day business trip to China with his father (an ambitious undertaking!). Before he left, the doctor made sure he was well stabilized with lithium and Lamictal and had an adequate supply. The doctor also prescribed Ativan (lorazepam) for anxiety or as a general calming medication to use "as needed," although they didn't end up using it. *"Did he complete the small amount of schoolwork I sent? No. Did he have jet lag? Yes, but not any worse than my husband. He was able to 'go with the flow' of my husband's business schedule and was able to stay back in the hotel one day when he was tired, tending to his lunch needs within the hotel and doing some schoolwork."*
- *Know what you need and be prepared:* In general, choose trips that are short or places you know well enough to anticipate what you need to bring and any issues that may come up. *"I make each child a gallon-sized snack bag with all their favorite snacks. It cuts down on those obsessive moments in the convenience store when you stop for gas."* Many parents keep comforting items (e.g., blanket, toy, doll, book, pillow, music) in the car or at their destination (such as Grandma's house); carry extra clothes; and make good use of electronic distractions, such as DVD players and video games.
- *Set ground rules:* Talk about the trip well in advance to help your child get ready for it. *"We explain the kind of rules and behavior that we expect, which are basically the same ground rules we have at home."*

- *Keep it low-key:* Many parents report that flexible, low-key, physically active vacations, such as camping, going to the beach, or hiking, work better than structured outings that involve a lot of public places, sightseeing, and long lines. These outdoor getaways allow the child to be a free spirit and expend her abundant energy: *"The girls can ride their bikes and meet camping friends, and we can get lots of fresh air and exercise."*
- *Have a back-up plan:* Be prepared to cancel, choose another event, separate the bipolar child from other children, or separate into two groups. *"If that doesn't work,"* said one parent, *"we leave no matter what."*
- *Maximize support:* You and your spouse should trade duties, go as a group with friends or family members who are equipped to help out, or, as I mentioned earlier, bring along a well-trained babysitter.

Other Special Situations

Like any other child, your child will benefit greatly from participating in sports, summer camps, and school trips and outings. With some extra effort and vigilance on your part, it is possible for your child to take advantage of these important life experiences, which will pay off in a number of ways if you can bypass some of the pitfalls. For instance:

Sports

Parents recognize that sports can be good for developing peer relationships and friendships, as well as for providing a physical outlet that helps moderate mood swings. As I have said earlier, however, non-team sports can be easier to negotiate for the bipolar child. Don't think your child has to excel at a sport in order to benefit. One parent whose child was on a swim team said, *"She doesn't get good coaching because she's obviously not good enough to ever win, but I don't care and I'm helping her not to care. She's made some friends and gets good exercise."* Pitfalls are many and include cruel peers or coaches and other adults (such as other parents, carpoolers, or chaperones) who do not understand and may unfairly criticize your child. In these cases, you'll have to take these adults aside to explain what works with your child, what doesn't, and why. Even if your child doesn't play on a team, being part of the experience can be beneficial. For example, one bipolar child helps his parents coach his 8-year-old sibling's team. *"He really feels good about being the 'assistant coach.'"*

Camps

You may think that day camps are out of the question for your bipolar child, but many parents have found suitable options in their communities. One child has been in a regular park district day camp for 6 years now, thanks to a one-on-one aide provided each summer (usually a psychology student for whom this experience is especially valuable). *"With the aide in place, Peter can participate as fully as he wants to, but if he needs to go off on his own or just wants to 'sit out,' he has someone with him,"* Peter's mother explains. *"The aide also acts as an explainer and mediator between Peter and the other kids, helping them understand him and vice versa."* There are special overnight camps that serve children with special needs, such as ADHD, mild ODD, and mild mood disorders. They provide structure, a low staff-to-camper ratio, and medication management. Some parents report difficulty transitioning to home after this kind of outing but feel that it was worth it because *"having as much normalcy as possible has been the best for her."* Also there is a quirk to bipolar children and especially teens. They are at times worse at home due to the intense relationships they generate, but act perfectly normally at camp, at times for 2 months in a row. They just manage low-emotion generic environments better than at home. I am open-minded and go on a case-by-case basis in deciding the best fit and comfort level.

Field Trips

If your child is going on a school trip, it is a good idea for a parent to go as a chaperone. If that's not possible, provide a letter to help explain to the group leader what to do if there is a problem. Sometimes it is difficult to keep a low profile and avoid calling attention to your child's problem. One mother advises, "Kids have to be taught to advocate for themselves and know how to speak up and get help if someone is perpetrating unfair or unkind treatment toward them due to stigma, or just creating unnecessary stress from meanness." It is up to you whether you share private information with other parents or teachers.

For more information and ideas, check out the website of the National Association of Therapeutic Schools and Programs (NATSAP;

www.natsap.org), which provides information about special schools, camps, and other programs and services appropriate for children with bipolar disorder and other mental illnesses.

Taking the Lessons to School

With greater peace and security at home, along with a comfortable routine including a good night's sleep, your child will be better prepared to cope with the larger, more unforgiving world, which includes school. In the next chapter, I will explain how you can apply many of these same lessons to the school setting, so your child can have a more positive, successful experience that paves the way for a successful life.

NINE

Finding the Best School Setting and Programs for Your Child

"Until we went through testing and evaluation, I never realized that brain-based learning problems are often part and parcel of the disorder. It helped me understand that my child needed help in schoolwork, especially math and reading."

"My daughter needs to go to the bathroom more often due to lithium, but the teacher wouldn't give her more breaks."

As a microcosm of the larger world, the school environment goes a long way toward shaping a child's self-esteem and success in life. This is especially true for a child with bipolar disorder, whose self-image is greatly affected by his or her interactions with peers, teachers, and other authority figures. In addition to creating social problems, your child's mood swings can affect his or her ability to think, pay attention, and learn. That may be why children with bipolar disorder often experience problems with reading and math and other difficulties processing information. We're discovering that their brains are "wired" differently in so many ways! It can be like your child is carrying heavy stones in his or her backpack that other children don't have, making school all the more challenging.

I don't wish to alarm you, but I do want to stress that lightening your child's "backpack load" and making it easier to function at school is absolutely critical to his or her development on every level—socially, emotionally, *and* intellectually. Although schools are required by law to help children with special social and learning difficulties, you play an important role in making sure that your bipolar child gets everything he or she needs. There are many well-trained and sincere people working in schools, but, like many healthcare professionals who have yet to catch up on advancing science, they may not understand or accept bipolar disorder and all the ways it could affect your child's school experience. Your job is to help educate them about your child's needs, encourage them to be compassionate, and direct the right resources to your child.

Considering how difficult things can be at home, you might have difficulty imagining your bipolar child coping at school without you there to help. At the same time, you might be glad that for 8 hours a day your child is in someone else's hands and, in fact, might do better with a teacher, who can stay more detached.

The primary goal is to make school a secure and safe environment by building the strengths of the child rather than dissecting behaviors and approaching each minor problem in school as a major obstacle. Working on problems collaboratively, involving the child in the process, and giving him or her choices in the classroom (within reason) will help your child blossom in ways you might not have thought possible!

Working with the School System

Getting the school working for your child can seem pretty daunting, especially if you're not familiar with how the system works. Whether private or public, schools are full of procedures, processes, and layers of bureaucracy. On top of that, they usually have too little funding to meet the needs of every student—a refrain you are likely to hear loudly and often. But if you come armed with knowledge about how the system works and what your child is entitled to receive under the law, you can make substantial progress. All it takes is a combination of planning, persistence, and patience, along with faith in your ability to make a difference for your child. You might feel like you are starting out at a disadvantage, particularly if your child has been having outbursts in the classroom or difficulty getting schoolwork done for some time. She may be unpopular with peers and viewed by teachers as a "problem student" because of disruptive behavior. You may not want to compound the problem by making waves, but it is important that you try to work with these important figures in your child's life, remembering that they are people with strengths, limitations, and personalities of their own. Teachers *are* in a powerful position to influence your child's life; therefore, I cannot overemphasize the importance of getting them on your side at the outset (see Chapter 10).

Your Child's Rights under Federal Law

Universal education is the cornerstone of American democracy. Our government guarantees that all children receive a "free and appropriate" education regardless of race, creed, color, gender, income, religion, or disability. For children with bipolar disorder and other mental illnesses, these basic educational rights are protected by the Individuals with Disabilities Education Act (IDEA) and Section 504 of the Rehabilitation Act.

Accessing Services

Determining how to go about accessing services under these laws—whether to use IDEA or file for Section 504—will depend on your child's specific needs, where you are in the United States, and what your particular school has to offer.

While the 504 plan may be enough for some children with milder illness, it may not offer quite enough for the child with full-blown bipolar

---

Educational Rights Websites

The following websites offer information on your child's legal right to an education and the processes for applying for accommodations or special education:

Technical Assistance Alliance for Parent Centers (funded by the U.S. Department of Education) (*www.taalliance.org*)
States' Protection and Advocacy Systems (*www.napas.org*)
Child and Adolescent Bipolar Foundation Educational Advocacy Center (*www.bpkids.org*)
Children and Adults with Attention-Deficit/Hyperactivity Disorder (CHADD) (*www.chadd.org*)

See the Resources for additional information on parent education and advocacy.

disorder, whose condition affects health *and* learning on so many levels. If your child's mood fluctuations and learning challenges continue to interfere with her school functioning despite appropriate medication and 504-style accommodations, she will probably need special education services under IDEA.

Be aware that Section 504 has fewer rules and regulations compared to those required by IDEA for an individualized education plan (IEP), which is a written document that outlines the supports and services the school agrees to provide for a child who is eligible for special education services. For instance, Section 504 does not discuss the role of outside evaluations, limit the frequency of testing, or require parental consent for testing. In addition, Section 504 does not require that an evaluation be conducted before a child receives a 504 plan or before making alterations to the plan. Because safeguards are less strict under Section 504, situations may arise that the plan won't cover. For instance, this may include a "stay-put" provision to maintain your child in his current environment while any issues are being resolved or having the plan travel with your child through the grades. (The box on page 198 sums up the salient differences between Section 504 accommodations and IEPs.)

As eager as you may be to use these laws to help your child get everything she needs, you do not have carte blanche to make unreasonable demands on the school system. We all want the very best education for our children, but that's not what these laws guarantee. They simply provide the resources needed to even the playing field for the child with disabilities and make sure she has the same opportunities to learn as her nondisabled peers. The single most useful resource to have in preparing for an IEP meeting is sample education plans from the CABF website to see how specific needs are matched with resources in reading, math, handwriting, speech therapy, occupational therapy, and counseling, along with planned time-outs. There are preplanned, formatted letters that you can sign and present to the school to begin the process. Please be aware, however, that the laws apply only to public schools. If your child is in private school, things often fall apart rapidly as problems exceed resources.

When Accommodations Aren't Enough

Some parents want their child to be accommodated in the regular classroom no matter what because it makes them feel that their child is "nor-

Should You Be Afraid of "Labeling"?

You might be concerned that your child will be "labeled" and ostracized if it becomes known that he has bipolar disorder. Parents are often advised by well-meaning friends that hiding their child's problem is the best course of action. But in this day and age, there are many kids with identified special needs, and it is much less stigmatizing than it was when we went to school a generation ago. The best thing you can do to improve his self-esteem is to give him the tools and support to succeed socially as well as academically. He may already judge himself very harshly, asking himself, "What's wrong with me?" or "Why don't people like me?" He may have scared away other children and already eats lunch alone. He may even think that his teachers "hate" him because of their increasing frustration with his behavior. Acknowledging that your child has a disorder that is not his fault can lift a heavy burden off his shoulders and yours. Explain that everyone has challenges in life—if not now, then later. It can also help teachers and other school staff be more compassionate and understanding of your child's situation, while it frees up more resources from the general education program, Section 504, or IDEA special education.

Some children don't mind being public about their battle with bipolar disorder. They may be idealistic and want to change the way people think about mental disorders by writing an essay or speaking in front of the class about it. One parent said, "In seventh grade, my son had a group assignment to make a presentation about an illness. He and his group chose bipolar disorder so that the other kids in his class could have a better understanding of his illness, to reduce stigma and misunderstanding. It was very well received." If they really want to do it, I recommend letting them unless there is a clear risk of abuse.

Of course, it should be up to you and your child how much information you want to share and with whom. You have the right to expect that the school will respect your child's privacy and keep his diagnosis confidential. The school may not release it to anyone outside the school system without your permission. Within the school, you also should be able to count on teachers and other school professionals to be discreet and not talk about your child loosely or call undue attention to your child's social and learning needs in front of peers or staff. Mind you, this may not be your experience, and I completely agree that, at times, any news about the disorder spreads like wildfire to all teachers and, before long, your child is branded. Don't panic! We can subdue this by gently making a clear request that you prefer teachers to treat the information discreetly and explain your fears. Your logic-based appeal will hopefully make an impression on the school team. This can generate some compassion and get the teachers to tune in to you. (More on forming an effective collaboration with your child's teachers is in the following chapter.)

mal." They also believe their child will learn more when mainstreamed with his peers. But other factors must be considered when choosing the right educational setting, including the severity of your child's problems, the kind of assistance available at the school, and the kind of treatment your child receives from peers. In some situations, a therapeutic school might be the best choice to maximize learning potential, access more individualized attention and tailored treatment, and establish better relationships with peers. I am all for normalizing, but not at the cost of a child's emotional well-being. If a child is being neglected or ostracized or is under too much stress, I usually recommend a well-operated therapeutic school. To find out more about special schools available in your area and how to go about choosing a specialized educational setting, see the website of the National Association of Therapeutic Schools and Programs (NATSAP) (*www.natsap.org*).

Getting Your School to Help

As parents, we often find ourselves automatically placed in the role of advocate for our child's education, yet we may feel overwhelmed or unequipped to navigate the maze of laws, services, and specialists. Fortunately, most school districts and state education offices have developed material to help parents become better informed about services and how to utilize them. There are also many independent parent support and advocacy groups that offer printed material, web-based resources, workshops, and phone consultation. See the Resources for more information.

Where to Begin

No matter where you live, the process of obtaining special services usually begins with either you or the teacher. It's not uncommon for the teacher to be the first one to spot a problem. In fact, it may be a particularly alert teacher who first spots a pattern of behavior—perhaps she noticed your child's rapid cycling of high and low moods or the perpetual inattention and distractibility associated with mood swings—that leads to your child being evaluated and diagnosed in the first place. But, as you're reading a book for parents of children with bipolar disorder, let's assume your child has already been diagnosed and you are now pursuing getting the child whatever school help he needs. These are some of the initial actions that other parents have found helpful:

1. **Prepare yourself mentally.** It can be hard to steel yourself to take on a large and complex institution like the schools. You may be weary and feel like you've already fought far too many wars—with the health-care system, with well-meaning family members, maybe even with your spouse—just to get a correct diagnosis for your child. You are on your own. Despite your fatigue, it is very important that you approach the schools in a calm, neutral, and businesslike manner. Dress nicely and maintain your poise, even if you're feeling less than confident to start with. You can also provide the school with copies of brochures or other literature about bipolar disorder so they can have a better understanding of the illness (see *www.bpkids.org* to request copies). There can be many delays, obstacles, and hurdles to get over, so save your energy and don't overreact—it will just hurt your case. Taking an experienced parent with you who can support you in negotiating with the school can make a big difference here. Another parent can not only help articulate your child's needs, she can also give you the moral support and understanding you need to carry on.

2. **Meet with the teacher.** If your child is in elementary school, make an appointment to talk with the classroom teacher to explain your child's condition and how it might affect behavior, peer relationships, and learning. If the teacher initiates the meeting, it may put you on the defensive, thinking that she is criticizing your parenting ability. Don't take it person-ally. You both have your child's best interests at heart, so work on the problem together. Don't make the mistake of skipping over the teacher and requesting an appointment with the principal. It undermines the per-son on the front line, and you don't want to anger her. The teacher will play a key role in both planning and implementing any accommodations your child gets, so it's critical to develop a plan together and forge an alli-ance with her right now. In middle or high school, make an appointment with your child's homeroom teacher or the school counselor assigned to your child. You might also meet with teachers for subjects that are most problematic for your child to devise a course of action together. Look at them as well-meaning individuals and put your best foot forward!

3. **If necessary, seek a higher authority.** If the teacher is not respon-sive to expressed concerns and you have tried everything else (see later in this chapter on developing a working relationship with the teacher), you

might need to contact the principal or director of special education directly. Again, be sure you've exhausted your options before going over the teacher's head. Mind you, we occasionally encounter a stubborn teacher or a complaining and punitive sort. Why should teachers be perfect as a population any more than the rest of us? In those cases, I often end up giving pep talks to children (and parents) that no one is perfect, but that they should try to change the things they can and live with the rest.

4. **Work out an interim plan.** In most localities, the principal makes a referral to a special team in the school, referred to as the School Support Team, Pupil Support Team, or Student Support Team (the name varies from district to district). This group is assigned to work out an intermediate plan of action that may include more observation, evaluation, temporary services, etc. These teams do not exist in every school, but they must be available *by law* at least at the district level. If you decide to talk to the local school district, however, first go to your child's teacher and/or school administrators to find out how to contact the district 504 coordinators, as each school district handles 504 plans differently. Section 504 accommodations are often put in place while an IEP is being developed if it turns out your child needs more than 504 help.

5. **Get an evaluation.** After some specified period of time, the team may make a referral to special education services for testing and evaluation. In most cases, these evaluations determine whether your child qualifies for services at all. If the child's bipolar disorder (or other disability) adversely affects her educational achievement, she should qualify under IDEA, in which case the school district is obligated by law to conduct a formal evaluation that should lead to the development of an IEP. If your child needs some kind of assistance but not necessarily special education services, she may qualify for the lesser services allowed under Section 504, but you may have to apply for those to get the ball rolling as the school district is not obligated to perform an evaluation in such cases. In some situations, you may have to work directly with the district's director of special education or whomever the principal suggests. Go in well prepared with your knowledge of the IDEA and Section 504 laws so that you are not put off by misstatements or misinformation (e.g., "I am so sorry, we don't have any testing slots until next school year"). You might even come prepared with an independent evaluation that you have paid for, but remember, only the school can determine if your child qualifies for accommodations. You can assist this process with a letter from your child's

doctor or therapist, but you still have to go through the school's procedures to confirm that your child qualifies for Section 504 or IDEA assistance.

6. **Know your rights.** To make sure you fully understand your district's 504 procedures (they vary), ask for a copy of your district's Policies
and Procedures on Section 504. This document may be referred to by var-

Section 504 Accommodations versus an IEP

Section 504	IEP (IDEA)
Safeguards civil rights of the disabled in all areas of life, including transportation, employment, and public access as well as education for the whole lifespan	Covers only special education, ages 3–21 (preschool through graduation)
Does not provide for funding	Provides funding
School district not obligated to offer	School district obligated to identify and evaluate all children suspected of having disabilities
Student doesn't have to need special education	Student does have to need special education in some form
No formal evaluation by school required; information gathered from various "knowledgeable" sources	Formal multidisciplinary evaluation by school required; school may have to pay for outside evaluation if parents disagree with school's evaluation
Parents must be notified of accommodations planned but do not have to consent	Requires parent's informed written consent
Requires a plan	Requires an IEP
Provides accommodations within general education	Provides services via any combination of special and general education
Very general requirements for reevaluation and review	Very specific requirements for reevaluation and review

ious names, including Procedural Safeguards or Parental Rights. This document will inform you of your rights and responsibilities, along with the school's, for getting your child the accommodations he may need. (IEP procedures are discussed below.)

7. **If you're going to request a 504 plan (or any other accommodations), put it in writing.** You should date and sign a letter that explains the purpose of the request by indicating where the concerns and problem areas lie. Some schools have forms for these "request for referral" letters. Remember to make a copy of the letter for your files and, if possible, *personally* give the original to your child's school for its records. Upon delivery, the school is required to begin an evaluation process following strict and clearly defined guidelines if it hasn't already done so.

8. **Where to turn for more help:** As Section 504 is a civil rights law, you can contact either the local school district or your regional Office for Civil Rights of the U.S. Department of Education to learn more about your child's educational rights. (Check your local phone book or the Resources for contact information.) Before speaking to the school district, it would be helpful to read "Protecting Students with Disabilities: Frequently Asked Questions about Section 504 and the Education of Children with Disabilities," available at the U.S. Department of Education website (*www.ed.gov/about/offices/list/ocr/504faq.html*). IEPs are enforced by the Office of Special Education and Rehabilitative Services of the U.S. Department of Education.

9. **Request complete information.** Ask for a complete listing of the kinds of resources available from the school so you understand what's easily obtained and what you might have to take additional steps to secure for your child. If an alternative school is suggested, visit and make sure it will address your child's needs before agreeing to outplacement. You may even wish to bring in a specialized consultant to help you shop for such a program. A directory of educational consultants, social workers, counselors, and therapists who work in this area can be found on the NATSAP website (*www.natsap.org*).

Referral and Evaluation for an IEP

While waiting for the referral to the team responsible for special education, the school may be able to create a temporary action or intervention plan for your child. This is particularly important if the situation is urgent—for instance, if your child has become emotionally unstable, explosive, and unmanageable because the teacher has used coercive or confrontational techniques to try to manage your child's behavior. This referral will start a series of evaluations and tests, requiring your written consent. These tests are designed to determine your child's strengths, where the difficulties lie, what services your child needs, and what modifications are required to ensure she is able to function at school. *In the event that the school denies testing, under law you have the right to appeal the decision.*

Outside Evaluations

If you have the financial and other resources to be able to do so, get your own psychological, psychiatric, or educational evaluations. If you suspect that the school system does not have the expertise or resources to evaluate your child appropriately, it is well worth the expense. Schools do not have to take outside evaluations into account if they are able to evaluate the child in the school system. In my experience, if a child has not been tested by the school and an IEP takes place, a psychological assessment will be performed unless the school agrees to use previous outside tests. Schools frequently fall behind with special education testing and evaluation, which can delay your child getting the help he needs. Also, remember, school testing personnel work for the school, and it can be hard for an evaluator employed by the school to press it to provide resources he knows it lacks. Your own independent evaluations may give you leverage that you may not get if you rely only on the school's evaluation resources.

Getting an independent evaluation can be costly, and it may not be covered by insurance. Sometimes the school system will pay for the outside evaluation, but generally this happens only when you have some leverage exerted by a lawyer you have retained. I would not recommend taking such a step unless the situation is extremely bad; bringing legal action can polarize the situation and further delay your child getting help. Outside evaluations usually come with letters or statements from the evaluators to the school indicating the types of resources your child may need. Likewise, you may have medical reports or psychiatric or psychological evaluations that will be helpful for school personnel in making decisions about educational, counseling, and social resources for your child. Provide all of these to the school, with a cover letter from you, before the school evaluation begins if you already have them and as soon thereafter as possible if you don't.

Physician Teleconference

Scheduling a teleconference for your child's psychiatrist or other physician who is familiar with bipolar disorder with the special education director, the school principal, the social worker, class teachers, resources teachers, and other school professionals is a very effective way to bring medical expertise to the evaluation and planning process. Given the level of myth and misunderstanding about bipolar disorder, this teleconference gives the physician an opportunity to educate the school personnel and parents about the chronic and cyclical nature of the illness and how that may affect the child's learning and social development. It also alerts everyone about potential risks and how the illness impacts relationships and self-esteem, increasing the team's empathy for the child and reducing the potential that the child will be ostracized by both adults and other students. It helps ensure that the child's emotional needs are considered and provides suggestions for engaging in collaborative activities for building the child's self-image, including pep talks, buddy systems, and leadership tasks. See Appendix H for a detailed framework for a physician teleconference that we found useful.

Navigating an IEP

A team of qualified school professionals will review the completed evaluation and determine if your child meets the eligibility criteria for an IEP. You will then be notified in writing. If she does not meet the eligibility criteria for an IEP, you can appeal this decision. If she does meet the criteria, the next step is that you will be invited to an IEP meeting, where an IEP will be created with your input and assistance. By law, you are an equal member of the team. The entire IEP process, from the initial meeting to the evaluation to the actual IEP meeting, is highly regulated, with specified timetables as to how long each part of the process may take.

You will work together in the IEP meeting to identify your child's needs, as well as goals your child will be expected to achieve by the end of 1 year. The team determines what services will be needed to help your child meet the goals, where they will be delivered, by whom, and how frequently. You can agree or disagree with the final IEP recommendations, but ideally you and the rest of the team should try to come to consensus. You give your agreement by signing the IEP, which then proceeds as outlined. If you disagree, the law stipulates that you are entitled to "due process," which is discussed below. The law also requires that the team meet at least once a year to review progress and/or determine if the IEP needs to be changed to meet your child's changing needs.

Things That Might Be Included in an IEP for a Bipolar Child

1. Classroom interventions/assistance/aid
2. Therapeutic school
3. Residential placement (see the section on residential treatment centers in Chapter 6)
4. Suggestions to the school team (social worker, teacher) concerning ways to build the child's social skills and self-esteem, such as pep talks, buddy systems, and leadership assignments and even lesser accommodations, such as
5. RAINBOW therapy
6. Educational supports and services (occupational therapy, speech, social skills training)
7. Communication between family and school
8. Medication information
9. Specific classroom accommodations, such as need for unlimited water/bathroom breaks, the ability to leave the room for a unscheduled meeting with the school social worker, a beanbag chair or other relaxation device in the classroom, relaxed rules about arriving at school on time, etc.

What Is a Therapeutic Day School?

These are special schools specifically designed to address the needs of children with behavior and mood disorders, learning disabilities, and multiple diagnoses. They can provide the bipolar child with a supportive, flexible environment that may do a better job of accommodating her physical, emotional, and social needs and allows her to be with her family and friends the rest of the time.

Maximizing the IEP

1. *Don't settle for less when more is needed.* Now you have some knowledge of how to obtain school resources, and you may feel prepared to ask

for what your child needs. Be forewarned that at some point you are likely to hear: "We can't give everyone what you're asking; we'd go broke." It's easy to be swayed by this argument—no one wants to think that getting what his own child needs means depriving another child. In fact, the worst-case scenarios are those where the school does not even admit the child's needs! Federal law stipulates that certain requirements be fulfilled for children with disabilities. We all understand that schools are under-funded, but how are they ever going to get sufficient funding if parents don't stand up for their children's needs and rights?

So, instead of feeling like you are asking too much, think of it this way: by advocating for your child and requesting appropriate resources, you are helping the teachers, principals, and administration demonstrate that their students have needs that the state legislatures must support. By clearly articulating your child's needs, you give the superintendent infor-mation she can use to justify the yearly budget request. Maybe I can remind you here to put on your business hat and depersonalize this from the school faculty; instead, emphasize the needs of your child. As more and more parents like you stand up for their children, all children will be better served.

2. *You don't have to say yes to whatever is offered.* Sometimes school personnel will list a limited set of services and say, "this is all there is." Well, if that is true, and it is not appropriate or sufficient for your child, calmly say no—this is your right. Saying no will trigger due process for appealing the decision.

3. *Take along an experienced friend.* Remember, when you go into an IEP meeting, take someone with you who can help you explain your child's needs and personally support you; otherwise you'll be significantly outnumbered by school personnel. If you haven't gone to an IEP before, take a friend along who has been there, seen it, and done it, someone knowledgeable and effective who understands your child's needs and yours. A physician teleconference, explained above, is also a valuable source of support. If you are uncertain of anything, don't sign, and don't agree until you can go home, think about it, and talk with others if needed. If there are serious differences of opinion, you can retain an expe-rienced special education/disability rights lawyer to advise you. See Chap-ter 7 for more about advocating for your child.

4. *Keep copies of everything.* Once you get the proposed IEP from the team assigned to your child, and after you read these materials and factor them into your action plan, remember to file them! You are likely to need

them later. In the concise words of one parent, "DOCUMENT EVERY-THING!"

Appealing an IEP

"Due process" is established by law to protect the rights of the child and parents. If you and the school district cannot agree about your child's needs and the school services required, a hearing is scheduled with an impartial mediator. Each side presents its arguments and evidence, and the hearing officer makes a final determination about what the educational program should be, based on the provisions of IDEA law. School districts are required to give you a copy of the special education procedural safeguards (or parental rights statement) when an evaluation is first scheduled and each time an IEP meeting is held.

The school system must coordinate due process at no cost to you, which can be an expensive proposition. Therefore, it is often easier for the district to agree to provide a resource requested by a parent than to go through the cumbersome legal process. Here are some tips about how to make the most of the process:

• Get an outside medical opinion. An opinion from someone familiar with the bipolar child's special needs is essential for making your case. Despite the cost, this up-front expense will help save money in the long run, once the school system begins to provide support you once had to pay for on your own.

• Consider compromising. You don't need enemies, particularly among people who spend every weekday with your child. You might agree to revisit currently denied service at the next IEP meeting. It's a good idea to put it in writing that if your child's school experience doesn't improve in a specific period of time, additional resources will be provided.

• Be polite, concerned, calm, and understanding, but be firm. The law specifies that children with mental illness are entitled to the resources they need to give them equal opportunity for educational success. If you believe something denied in the IEP is critical, stand by your convictions. Sometimes, school faculty may feel patronized if you bring up the "the law says" cliché over and over, but negotiating tangible solutions while working out the bottom line of getting what your child needs is important.

• Even if you feel like you've hit a dead end, don't give up. One mother tried to get all resources available from the school in a normal classroom, starting with an aide. With much prodding, the school provided 1 hour of help per day. This was adequate the first year, but things got tougher in the second year, and the aide changed. The new aide was inexperienced. Knowing that a very sensitive bipolar child can react to this rather critical simplistic teaching aid, it is not surprising that things fell apart. The school absolutely refused to pay for the resources. Although the mother was generally very diplomatic and the teacher was kind, the principal would not budge, feeling the school had given the child what was needed. The mother then called the director of the board of education directly and lobbied for her case. As a result, the school not only replaced the aide but also provided additional tutoring 3 days a week.

What If Your Child Is Having Significant Struggles at School?

Sometimes, no matter how hard you work with your school system, your child's needs cannot be met in a regular school environment. Social problems, learning problems, behavioral difficulties, and the resulting impact on self-esteem may be too great.

A good example was Matthew, a handsome, blond, blue-eyed 10-year-old treated in our clinic. His mother tried to get an evaluation through his school, but the simple psychological testing provided as part of "due process" underestimated his needs, and the school merely supplied additional tutoring in math. In reality, Matthew was unable to cope with school in many areas and at many levels. His comprehension, problem-solving, and planning abilities were very poor. He was distractible and impulsive, but stimulants worsened his mania. He had violent suicidal impulses whenever he could not solve a math problem, when the teacher singled him out for additional help, or when he felt criticized. His overly sensitive nature scared the teachers. When he showed his distress by trying to cut his wrists, the school refused to keep Matthew in the classroom. We then arranged for extensive independent neuropsychological testing and discovered that he had attention deficits, working memory deficits, and executive function problems. Despite thorough medical testing and a stable regime, he could not cope with these psychological problems coupled with his complicated and fragile sense of self.

Despite initial resistance, his mother agreed to deviate from "normal schooling" and allowed the school system to place him in a therapeutic day school. Matthew is currently thriving, and he is slowly mustering his internal strength, as external pressures and feelings of academic failure have been removed. Sometimes, truly, therapeutic schools are a blessing. Remember to shop for the right fit before you settle on one choice, as some schools will be set up for children with behavior and conduct disorders, and their approach to behavior management may not be suitable for a bipolar child!

Parents often resist the idea of placing their child in a special program or therapeutic school. They understandably don't want to take the child out of a familiar classroom or school, away from family members and friends whom the child may rely upon. They may also have idealized notions about mainstreaming their child and keeping the family together at all costs. They may feel like a failure, or like they've given up on their child, if they consider these options. Deciding when to stop trying to handle things on your own is difficult. We have placed a number of these children in residential treatment facilities with remarkable changes for the better. If resources allow, these are important alternatives to consider.

Cultivating a Good Working Relationship with School Staff

When things go wrong, you're much more likely to get them going right again quickly when you've laid the groundwork for a fruitful alliance with your child's school.

- *It all starts with good relationships with school staff.* In most cases, the people you have to deal with are just like you: they want to do a good job and feel appreciated for it, and they usually give it their best effort. If they feel attacked, they will become defensive and feel justified in rejecting your requests. As they are likely giving up lunch or another mealtime to meet with you, bringing food (muffins for early morning meetings or cookies for a mid-afternoon meeting) will help make them more receptive. It's like the adage says: You can catch more flies with honey than with vinegar.
- *Understand the school system's limitations.* Try to empathize with school personnel and understand that they have a difficult job, are underpaid to do it, and have too few resources to work with. When

you press for additional assistance for your child, you may not be making their day any easier. So look for ways to avoid win–lose interactions. Whenever possible, create win–win strategies. For example, you win when you obtain the necessary additional resources your child needs, and school personnel also win when they feel understood and appreciated for going the extra mile to help your child.

- *Get to know the school nurse.* Your child's health and safety are a great concern, particularly if your child's disorder causes her to behave aggressively toward other children or threaten to harm herself. The school nurse can be a great resource for looking after your child's physical and emotional well-being and offer a safe harbor if your child needs a time-out to deal with a mood change.
- *Pick your battles carefully.* If you are not sure something is worth fighting for and feel stressed about it, set it aside for a week or two. Don't even think about it if you can avoid it. Then revisit the issue. Was it worth the energy you were expending? Is it still worth it? Does your best friend agree? Do other experienced parents agree? If not, let it go and move on. But if that is impossible—if you *still* feel too strongly—set it aside for another 2 weeks.
- *Anticipate problems and offer solutions.* This is an important strategy that will make it easier to create win–win solutions that others feel good about. It can be hard to predict the future, but, as you talk with others and gain personal experience, you'll be better able to project what is likely to go wrong. For instance, you might be feeling anxious about the fact that a new teacher is scheduled to start in the middle of the year. Will she be willing to work with you in nurturing the child's interests with the plan that seemed to be going well, or will she insist on her own system? At the next IEP meeting, you can bring up this concern and ask how to ensure that the school cooperates with you in using positive interpersonal strategies (more on this below). But put yourself in the school staff's shoes for a minute—how could you help them make the transition as painless as possible? Perhaps you could suggest setting up a meeting with the new teacher before she starts to tell her a little about your child, describe the difficulties of a bipolar child and how you negotiate with him, and see if the teacher is agreeable to using a compassion-driven yet firm approach instead of consequence-based behavior modification. This way, you serve as a

liaison between school staff, your child, and your child's therapist. You directly influence staff's behavior, which benefits staff as well as your child.

- *Act early and act fast.* Work early in the year with the principal to form a good relationship with her. That way, when you want to start planning for next year, you've already got a strong ally. Don't hesitate to do some detective work early in each school year. As you hook up with other parents, find out from them who the best teachers are for the next year. If you don't know this by now, you only have to experience it once to know that a given teacher, one that your child likes and thinks likes him, can make a *huge* difference in your life and your child's.

- *Document your reasons for requesting a service or change for your child.* Write up your ideas for services that need to be added or changed and ask your family physician to send it with his own cover letter supporting your request. This approach can go a long way toward having the school take your ideas seriously.

- *Join the PTA.* Get involved in whatever parent association or other group is available. Being active on special education committees can be especially helpful. If you are the only one who is causing problems for the school system, you'll have much less leverage than if you speak with and for the PTA or a group of other parents. Identify other parents whose children have similar needs and, when appropriate, organize them to present concerns. Even if it's only three or four of you, the input of multiple parents is a powerful force, and keeping parents happy is central to any administrator retaining his job and making the school board members happy.

- *Volunteer to help.* Whether it's in the classroom itself, the library, or the front office, being seen and becoming known as a regular and positive presence at the school makes you an insider. It helps make you part of the solution, not part of the problem, and positions you as an ally rather than an adversary. This strategy has the further advantage of giving you the opportunity to observe your child's behavior more directly. One mother said volunteering in her child's class once a week improved her communication with the teachers. She got to know them better, understand what went on in class, and see their interactions with her child and others. You can also help alleviate the teacher's stress by volunteering to do something which frees up her time to work with your child and others who might need extra help. Chaperoning field trips, working school fund raisers, or helping secure additional resources such as furniture and computers are all effective ways to increase teachers' ability to assist children with special needs in the classroom. Often, parents who have been beaten down by the illness can become bitter and resentful. Keep a positive attitude—being helpful and pleasant will help your child have a better school experience.

Troubleshooting School Barriers

Parents often feel as if their job is done once an IEP or Section 504 plan is finally in place, but bipolar disorder is chronic and cyclical and can change over time. Breakthrough symptoms come and go. What do you do when new problems arise? What if a particular teacher is unable to empathize or deal appropriately with your child's mood fluctuations? What if a medication change produces a crisis in the classroom? The following tips should prove useful:

- Speak candidly and confidentially to the principal, and ask for his advice. Asking for help and putting others in a position to help you, rather than leaving them to feel you are demanding something of them, is often a wise strategy.
- Get a sense from other parents of the tenor of an unsympathetic teacher's reactions in general to the other kids in the classroom; revisit the situation with your doctor, who can write a letter or conduct a teleconference with the professionals involved to diffuse the tension and overcome the barriers.
- Whom do you know on the school board? Talk with them. This is generally useful if you need to address broader issues of changing rules or getting insight into school faculty and their systems.
- There is strength in numbers; enlist other parents' support and approach the school collectively. Find out about good strategies from the PTA, local parent groups, or CABF and NAMI. What have other experienced parents done that has worked?
- Go to the superintendent and request alternative arrangements such as residential placement. Be aware that, unless your child is experiencing psychosis, has a severe conduct disorder, or has had

multiple hospitalizations, it is next to impossible to get your child into a residential facility for free.

- As a last resort, send a letter from your lawyer. There are lawyers who are expert at this. CABF or other parent groups may be able to make a referral to someone experienced in this area. But really use legal leverage as a last resort—picking battles with the school over every little issue will cause the school to tune you out and limit your ability to make headway on the really important issues.

Sometimes the battle isn't worth it. Is there another school that you can transfer your child to? A therapeutic school? A residential center? NATSAP provides information about these types of programs and the professional assistance available for selecting the right program to meet your child's educational and clinical needs.

The Teacher:
Your Child's Greatest Ally at School

I mentioned at the beginning of this chapter how important it is to create an alliance with your child's teacher. All the best school accommodations you can get for your son or daughter won't amount to much if you don't have a good working relationship with your child's teacher. The next chapter will help you establish a partnership with this critical person in your child's life.

TEN

Forming a Partnership with Your Child's Teacher

Your child's teacher(s) will make a big difference in the kind of day your child has at school. The most effective teachers for a child with bipolar disorder use a mix of patience, structure, positive discipline, consistency, and nurturance. If the teacher is compassionate and collaborative, involves your child in decisions, and gives him choices (within reason), it can be a good experience. If, on the other hand, the teacher is opposed to making accommodations or focuses on the negatives, makes an issue of minor infractions, uses punishment, and forces your child to cooperate, it can increase the intensity of the situation and cause your child to fight back. The majority of the time, bipolar children will need some type of accommodation (see Chapter 9 on how to obtain the help your child needs), and they typically respond better when adults discuss things ahead of crises and avoid power struggles.

What Kind of Teacher Is Best for Your Child?

Even some well-intentioned and kind teachers can come up short in the skills needed to work with the bipolar child in the classroom. Sometimes teachers skilled in working with students with special needs may get frustrated and exasperated and see your child as a discipline problem, rather than a child in crisis. That's why it's so important for you to help educate teachers and other professionals who deal with your child at school about the best behavior management strategies. Effective teachers of children with learning disabilities keep the children engaged in learning by using a varied, multisensory teaching style, getting responses from them, calling their names during instruction, using exciting examples and illustrations, and frequently praising them for cooperation and attention. How hard it is to get this kind of teaching for your child will depend on what you and the teacher are up against. If the student–teacher ratio in your child's school is low, the teachers are fairly knowledgeable about learning problems, and they seem genuinely dedicated to giving all their students an equal opportunity to learn, you're way ahead of the game.

If your child is involved in your school's special education program or at a specialized school, there should be at least a few teachers trained in learning and behavior problems. Whether your child has their assistance part-time or full-time, they can be a good resource within the school. A one-on-one tutor can be a great help in keeping up academically for students who suffer from anxiety and low self-esteem. The downside of this scenario is that your child may not get as many opportunities to socialize with peers who are at the same grade level, so you may have to work with the school to create chances for your child to mix with the general student population in a way that doesn't increase his anxiety. Special education teachers are not only talented and dedicated to helping special needs kids, but are trained in methods that allow them to attend to the necessary detail. In addition, in therapeutic and residential settings, your child will have the benefit of a low student–teacher ratio. These schools have extra resources with all types of therapists—psychologists, physiotherapists, occupational therapists, and those who offer aid in reading and writing. There are often nurses who sit in the classroom or are available at the drop of a hat. The whole environment is one of all-around supportive care and seasoned expertise. There is no one type or set of experts, however, that you can expect to find at every school. Each school will differ to some degree in staff and peer group according to its expertise. Some take cognitively typical but emotionally challenged kids, some take tough kids with behavior disorders, and some cater to cognitively challenged youth.

Partnering with Your Child's Teacher

The other ingredient you need to optimize your child's school experience is a productive partnership with teachers. A good partnership is even more critical when teachers have a large student load, are unfamiliar with bipolar disorder and related learning disorders, and are simply worn out by all the demands placed on them, including those from other parents. Regardless of the circumstances at the school, the education of children is a responsibility that must be *shared* by the teacher and parent as *partners*. Teachers need to recognize what a powerful asset a parent can be; parents need to appreciate how important teachers are to a child's success.

In my practice, I work with families on incorporating the RAIN-BOW tips into their daily lives (described in Chapter 6). Many of these principles can be very helpful in the school setting, helping teachers avoid problems and getting the family and school on the same page with respect to managing the bipolar child's behavior. Adapting the RAIN-BOW approach to the classroom includes educating the teacher about bipolar disorder, showing her how to monitor mood changes, and encouraging her to use collaborative problem solving and pep talks rather than punitive measures with your child.

What Else Teachers Can Do to Help

A teacher may have as many as 30 sets of parents to satisfy, and you are just one of them. What is reasonable to expect of teachers, and what is not?

Respond to Your Requests for Information about Your Child's Progress

As you know, regular times are set up throughout the school year for teachers to give parents feedback—in most schools anywhere from two to four conferences, more for younger children, and fewer as they get older. But those parent–teacher meetings are set up to serve as a *minimum* level of communication between you and the teacher. Your child has special needs, greater than many of the other children in the classroom, so close coordination is essential. You want to be able to give your child positive feedback for giving his best effort at school, and the only way to give that feedback soon enough for it to count is probably to confer with the teacher weekly—more often in crisis situations and less often, perhaps only monthly, when things are stable.

Set a Positive Tone

The teacher's attitude toward your child will affect the way other students view him and how he sees himself, so it is very important that you work with the teacher to gain understanding and acceptance from the very start. One bipolar child I know had a teacher who set a very demanding, rigid tone in the classroom. The child often came home thinking he was "stupid" and "dumb" for not keeping up and that "all the kids in my class hate me." "The teacher set the tone that my child was an outcast," the parent said. "He would have panic attacks because of the stress in that classroom."

Monitor and Reward Good Behavior

A very good technique for keeping the lines of communication open between home and school is the "Good Behavior Book." This tool can help teachers focus on your child's positive behavior and progress by highlighting at least three good things that happened during the week and sending that information home with the child. This will give you an opportunity to add your praise and hugs for good behavior.

The "daily report card" (DRC) is another convenient tool that can help teachers communicate with parents. The DRC is simply a sheet of paper on which the teacher rates the child's performance on an agreed-on small (four to five) set of target behaviors for the child. If there is a string of undesirable behavior with poor progress for days in a row, perhaps it is best to stop the DRC so as not to trigger rejection sensitivity. One important note: When you set up a reward system, very often, bipolar children get overenthusiastic and intense in their reward-seeking behavior, pushing to get their rewards sooner and sooner and talking about them nonstop. Thus, keeping it simple and in moderation is the rule.

Keep You Apprised of Homework Assignments

Along with the DRC, you may want to include a place for the teacher to note your child's homework assignments. Assignments might be written down in a little notebook by the child and initialed by the teacher. This way, the teacher does not have to write down each assignment for each child (increasingly hard to do as the number of children with special needs mounts). Instead, your child has this responsibility, along with the task of getting the teacher's signature or initials on what he has written down. Some teachers will give everyone a homework sheet, where assignments, particularly longer-term projects, are spelled out more clearly. This can be a lifesaver for bipolar children, who may have difficulty processing verbal instructions. One parent told how, when her daughter asked for clarification on verbal assignments, the teacher would answer, "Emily, what is the matter with you? Why don't you pay attention?" and, thus, her daughter stopped asking for clarification and doing the homework. In this case, you might suggest the teacher try providing written directions for your child, but be sure to ask whether the assignments lend themselves to it. Otherwise, from the teacher's perspective, you may be recommending more work for him.

Be Concerned

Your child's teacher should be genuinely concerned about and caring for your child and her progress. He should make your child feel welcome and liked in the classroom. How can you tell if this is the case? In many instances, the child will like the teacher because she feels valued and liked in return. If your child doesn't feel that way, it could mean that the teacher, however well intentioned, may not be communicating it effectively or may have said something that your child interpreted as a personal rejection. If you are convinced this is true, reassure your child that the teacher *does* like her. Give your child a little gift that she can give to the teacher to show that the teacher is valued for her hard work. Remember, we are all human beings and social beings who love to be liked and appreciated. If you think the teacher can hear the information and respond well, share your concerns with him. Sometimes teachers don't realize how thin-skinned bipolar children can be. Drawing it to their attention may encourage them to go out of their way to communicate their caring feelings for your child.

Sometimes you will sense that the teacher actually *does not* like your child. Children with special needs do add to a teacher's burden, and given the intensity of the bipolar child's personality and the potential for difficult behavior, some teachers may feel defensive, frustrated, helpless, or baffled by your child. If you sense a teacher's dislike, exasperation, or incompetence, your child probably does, too. Here you may have to try a number of strategies to see if you can change things around. The "apple for the teacher" trick might help. Sending the teacher thank-you notes or maybe even just getting together to commiserate could make a difference. If the teacher is aloof or curt with all children, it could be tougher to turn around, but, in this scenario, at least you can feel your child is not the only victim. It could even be an opportunity to teach your child that all people are different, with different strengths and weaknesses, and even teachers can get moody.

Avoid Punitive Approaches with Your Child

Schools at times have been more punitive than positive. Your child's teachers may have more experience with children who have ADHD than those with bipolar disorder, but techniques that work with ADHD can potentially backfire with the bipolar child, causing him to avoid class or become defiant or stubborn. One parent laments that her child never earns "free-time Friday" because she never does her homework, yet she has an accommodation for no homework on her IEP. "How is that fair?" Unduly or frequently restricting recess, berating your child, drawing negative attention to him in front of the class, and assigning tedious make-work tasks intended to be corrective behavior are all counterproductive with the bipolar child and can set off an unnecessary power struggle. You know better than the teacher how difficult your bipolar child can be to handle, but you also know that punitive approaches coupled with a poor teacher–child relationship are an explosive combination. Pep talks, keeping the Good Behavior Book, and other collaborative techniques can produce much better results.

Make Any Necessary Classroom Accommodations

Accommodations should be aimed at counteracting your child's difficulties to make her school day work out better. These can include seating arrangements, homework accommodations, a system to inform you of the day's assignments, more frequent bathroom breaks, and chances to take a time-out in the nurse's office. For one child, a spot was made in a small room near his class where he could go until he calmed down. An adult stayed with him but gave him no attention because any stimulation would make the meltdown worse. The school kept a basket of fidget toys handy both in the classroom and in the child's "meltdown place" because they were calming for him. If you get the impression that your child's teachers and other school staff may not be familiar with the techniques that work best with bipolar children, you can suggest some of the positive techniques you use at home. Remember, if you want the teacher to be willing to work with you, these should be posed as *suggestions*, not demands. Also, keep in mind that not all techniques will work with every child, so you should look for opportunities to help the teacher identify modifications and accommodations that work for your child based on previous experience.

Put in at Least a Little Extra Time

There's no question that accommodating a child with bipolar disorder adds to the teacher's workload, but it is required by law. The time and effort needed to provide your child with necessary accommodations shouldn't mean that your child gets cheated in other areas. You can suggest ways to keep the teacher's additional time investment to a minimum, such as using a positive note exchange or having your child write the homework assignments down, with the teacher needing only to initial the page. Remember, when you're asking a teacher to put in a *little* extra time, you're not asking for the moon. Be sure to show your appreciation to the teachers who take it upon themselves to go the extra mile every day.

Occasionally, teachers will make helping your child a personal mission. They sincerely want to help but may not understand what they have taken on. "He is a charming kid, so teachers are willing to go out of their way, but then they get frustrated and get mad at him for 'not helping himself,'" said one parent. "I've watched so many teachers go from 'I'm going to be the one to make him a success' to 'I'm fed up with him and will treat him hard.' Neither approach has worked." You may need to step in and help well-meaning teachers understand your child's limitations before their good intentions turn to disappointment for both your child and them.

How to Get the Teacher on Your Side

As a parent, you can expect and receive cooperation from most teachers by appreciating and relying on their expertise, recognizing how hard their job is, and informing them about what your child needs and responds well to. You can help teachers understand and nurture your child. Most teachers don't know a lot about pediatric bipolar disorder (many doctors don't either!), and they aren't trained to work specifically with bipolar children. Like some doctors, some teachers may not even take it seriously, preferring to think that your child is just "too sensitive" or "out of control." You play a very important role in educating them about the nature of the disorder and the difference between it and a learning disability such as ADHD or a behavior disorder such as a conduct disorder. You can order brochures from the Child and Adolescent Bipolar Foundation at *www.bpkids.org* specifically designed to educate teachers about bipolar disorder. You can also help teachers recognize symptoms of an impending relapse by familiarizing them with the behaviors listed in the Child Mania Rating Scale—Teacher Version (without actually asking the teachers to use the scale to rate the child; see Appendix C for a copy of this tool).

Always approach teachers and school personnel in an open, non-defensive, yet assertive way. Most of them really want to do the best job possible, despite often being overwhelmed. As a result, you must also show your appreciation to the teacher and the school when they do something well. Bringing in baked goodies, sending thank-you notes, remembering teachers' birthdays, and volunteering to help out on school trips are just some of the ways you can forge a good relationship with teachers.

Making the Partnership Work

In every interaction with the child's teacher, you can be actively building an effective partnership. To make that partnership work, you should:

- Reduce any anxiety your child might have about the coming year by having a planning meeting with a new teacher ahead of time.
- Communicate your concern from the beginning of the school year. Sit down with your child's teachers to talk about bipolar disorder and explain strategies that have been effective for him in school in the past.
- Establish positive, frequent communication. Drop the teacher a note telling him how much you appreciate him when you see any positive effort on his part. Make sure he knows you, likes you, and wants to go out of his way for you.
- Ask parents whose children had this teacher last year what kinds of approaches worked best with this particular teacher.
- Consider using a note pad to communicate success, concerns, or skills to work on on a weekly basis.
- Take every opportunity to show that you appreciate the teacher. For example, find out her birthday and have your child bring a small gift to class. Bring in a cake on that day and lead the kids in

singing "Happy Birthday." Or bake cookies for her and the class on Valentine's Day.

- Keep the teacher informed of any important changes in your child's life or treatment, especially any medication changes that could affect his behavior in class. If you have found a technique that seems to work particularly well, share it with him. He may want to apply it as well. If your child is upset and bothered about something, let the teacher know so he can anticipate any new behavior or mood problems and respond in a helpful manner.
- Talk to the teacher at the first sign of a problem and alert her to the signs of an impending mood change.
- Make school behavior and academic success part of your child's reward program at home, based on entries in the Good Behavior Book or frequent positive notes sent home by the teacher.
- How about asking the teacher what you could do to make her life easier? Maybe offer to volunteer in some way that has nothing to do with your child. Perhaps the teacher needs help coaching kids in the classroom in their writing projects, and that might free her up to do something that you'll want for your own child later.
- Ask the teacher if he needs any supplies for the classroom. We hear more and more about how teachers spend their own money on supplies or depend on donations from parents for things large and small.

As partnerships grow, trust also grows, and it may be appropriate and useful for you to share information with the teacher not just about your child, but also about the larger issues with pediatric bipolar disorder. As you get more expert, it is very likely that you may know more about what kinds of classroom strategies work and don't work for your child. Here are a few tips you can share that incorporate concepts of RAINBOW therapy as well as other practical technique.

You could give your child's teachers the tips as a handout, or you might want to find a more subtle, indirect way to pass them on. In my experience, teachers don't appreciate being told how to do their job any more than any other professional, but if you can make it perfectly clear that these tips are based on principles you've learned that help your child manage his behavior at home, you may gain a receptive audience. At the very least, you might find a chance to share the tips subtly on an as-needed basis, even if only one at a time.

10 Tips for Teachers Working with a Bipolar Child

1. Emphasize the positives. Instead of saying, "don't get out of your chair," say, "please sit down."
2. Praise more and criticize less. Make three positive statements for each negative comment. Use the Good Behavior Book to document positive behaviors and share them with parents.
3. Give simple, direct instructions, in writing if possible.
4. Decrease distraction.
5. Be calm and logical—don't "lecture."
6. Give the bipolar child leadership opportunities, such as taking attendance sheets to the office, cleaning the blackboard, or keeping the class calendar.
7. Give many opportunities for bathroom breaks, time-outs, and visits to the school nurse, and follow through on any other agreed-upon accommodations.
8. Reward good behavior with positive feedback rather than tangible objects.
9. Keep expectations realistic and tailored to the child's strengths.
10. Give frequent pep talks of 10 to 15 minutes one to seven times a week based on needs.

Teachers are very good at recommending other children who will be good friends for your child so you can arrange play dates. They will be an excellent resource to remind you of your child's particular strengths and interests as they spend a great deal of time with your child during the day.

Addressing Your Child's Social Needs

Stabilizing your child's school life is half the battle. Once school is under control and manageable for both you and your child, it's time to work on making life even better by helping your child develop satisfying friendships and other relationships. The next chapter deals with that all-important aspect of life.

ELEVEN

Building Social Skills
for Positive Friendships

"Last time I remember Andy being invited to a birthday party was 2 years ago. No one wants to be around him. He is so intense, loud, goofy, and before you know it, play fights turn into serious fights."

"Ellie is so friendly, so making friends is piece of cake. But keeping them is the real challenge. She is bossy and overpowering. Ellie feels betrayed, hurt, and angry but does not realize her role in driving away her friends."

How to Help Your Child Make and Keep Friends

Peer relationships are one of the most challenging areas for a child with bipolar disorder. They frequently have difficulty communicating with other children, are perceived as bossy or pushy (or irritable or shy), and have difficulty making and keeping friends. This leads to difficulties when they are at school, participating in extracurricular activities, or pursuing other social activities.

It is important to help your child learn to establish and maintain these essential peer relationships as so much of her future success and happiness depends on the ability to form lasting, satisfying bonds. **Feeling safe in a relationship is key to building intimate ties. Being appreciated is like cement bonding two people together.**

Although getting your home life and the school system in order will occupy much of your time and attention, it is also important to put energy into this area. Recognizing that it will be a process and take shape slowly, there's a lot you can do to help your bipolar child navigate this important but difficult aspect of life.

Identify the Right Friends: "Good Fit"

Friends come in all shapes and sizes! They are funny, serious, sweet, or witty. The key is finding those children who potentially "fit" well with your child—children who appreciate *and* enjoy spending time with your child. Look for compassionate personalities who demonstrate loyalty and willingness to play with your child. A true friend can be a godsend: "When our son has a problem, his friend just says, 'well, I have to go home for a bit.' An hour or two later they are back together." After a while, you can help your child spot these potential companions.

It may feel like you're trying to identify "willing victims" for your child—peers who will tolerate their excesses and roll with the punches (figuratively)—but don't feel guilty. With your supervision and teaching, the friend can be lucky to have play dates with your child. Make friends with the friends' parents at least to a degree that you can set up play dates or make a friendly phone call. Take a positive attitude—that you are offering something fun and valuable to the other child. Offering to pick up or drop off their child can help sweeten the deal for her parents.

It's a myth that so-called healthy kids know all about socializing and your child does not. Other children don't automatically have all the necessary skills to cope either; they are still young and developing, too, and may vary in their ability to interact, empathize, or exercise self-control. Don't expect too much. Even your child's closest friend can get fed up and impatient, as bipolar kids can be very (I mean *very*) *bossy*. They make rules and are intrusive. They want their way or walk off, call other kids "stupid," or swing a baseball bat at another child. It can get scary. Even adults can become aggravated if they have to face this kind of bossy behavior, so imagine another child trying to negotiate this loud, intrusive, demanding child. It takes a strong bond to withstand the ups and downs of these relationships.

It is really OK to tell the truth, such as that the play date was rough and you, too, were a bit upset, and then give your child a hug. You're expressing a genuine feeling in a moment of bonding. In sharing the pain, you gain intimacy with your child. So tell the truth, but remember that children can really hang on to feelings they know you share and might get obnoxious with that other kid. It's important later on to teach your child not to throw a stone into a dirty ditch, as an old saying goes, or she might get hit in the face with dirt. Teach your child to let it go.

Teach the Fine Art of Friendship

Like many things in life, friendship is a learned skill, especially for the bipolar child, who bounces between the two poles of extreme bossiness and extreme rejection sensitivity, often quite rapidly. This can make your child seem odd or obnoxious, limiting the willingness of other children to spend time with him. *"She is difficult to play with. She has to have control and is bossy. Kids don't like playing with her for too long. I always make sure I stay where she is playing so I can intervene if I have to."*

All kids want to have fun, be accepted, and have a good time, but when your child is intense, bossy, or reactive, it is super-hard for other children to take! It ruptures the pleasant expectations that kids come to play for. As a result, they may like your child but can't stand her. For example, 8-year-old Sam wanted Sarah to come play with her. Sam insisted Sarah paint her nails blue. Sarah liked coral, but she agreed reluctantly. Then Sam went on to put makeup on her. Sarah tried to refuse, as her mom does not approve. Sam insisted on using heavy makeup and then pushed Sarah to wear red lipstick. Sarah literally started to cry because she was afraid she would get into trouble with her mom. Sam's mom saw this occurring and gently asked Sarah if putting powder on her face might be OK, like face painting, and that she would explain to Sarah's mom about it on her behalf. She also explained to Sam that lipstick might be over the top for Sarah as they have different rules in their home. It was an agreeable middle solution. Furthermore, Sam's mom had a teaching moment with Sam that night about how to respect others' wishes and give them space.

Here's another common example. Aaron incessantly picks on peers. He suffers from such low self-esteem and a deep sense of insecurity, and he thinks the only way he can feel good about himself is by putting his peers down. He teases and taunts other children with remarks like "That is so dumb"; "How can you be so stupid?"; and "Oh my God, you are so bad at that." Can you, as a parent, teach your child better ways to get along with peers? Can your child be taught to stop pushing before a friend starts crying or coached to feel good about himself without making others feel bad?

As these examples show in part, your job is fourfold. First, help your child understand the process of making and keeping friends and explain how critical and bossy behavior interferes. Second, arrange appropriate play dates and create opportunities to learn and practice new relationship skills. Third, supervise, observe what is going on, and intervene directly and discreetly. Fourth and most important, build your child's self-esteem through praise and appreciation of the good things he does or says.

For example, one child was routinely ignored on the playground, and the other children wouldn't pass him the basketball. His mother coached him by saying, "Oh, *the only reason they don't pass you the ball is because they are afraid you'll show them up."* When the child did finally get the ball, he made a perfect basket. *"He never complains anymore now about the playground stuff,"* his mother said.

Your therapy program should be helping teach your child life skills for handling pressure and communicating feelings, which is an important part of building social relationships. You can proactively step in and teach your child how to manage these relationships before the situation escalates into continuing conflict or complete social isolation. This involves "priming" your child before the play date or social event, coaching him on ways to avoid becoming reactive or overly bossy. *"We rehearse social situations ahead of time,"* reports one mother. *"Even the simplest things like how to say hello to a classmate in the hallway at school."* Active teaching in an endearing manner will stick. Make sure you sound like you are on his side, but explain how to make things better for both parties—teach him "win–win" thinking. One parent sums it up this way: *"A healthy, positive mindset will get these kids through life. If they learn early on how to handle hurts, they will become strong, capable adults. Positive thinking is one of the best tools."*

Don't think of play dates as opportunities to leave the children alone and take a rest, as much as you deserve the break. One mother said that taking the time to lay a lot of positive groundwork when her child was young worked well for their family: *"We kept close supervision and tried to keep as many positive experiences and activities as possible, mixed with plenty of downtime to rest and regroup."* To the contrary, these social occasions can be very time consuming for you. Some children require constant one-on-one supervision, while others just need an occasional reminder. Either way, it's another project to set aside time for. If you recognize this, you will be less stressed. The idea is to discreetly hang around and give even more subtle feedback to influence "friend-friendly" thinking in your child.

Hopefully, after a while, you will be able to leave your child and her friends to play on their own.

While it looks like it is no big deal to correct your child in front of her friend, it can be pretty embarrassing. If there is an incident, debrief with the other child without putting your child down or pitting her against her guest, but be sure to empathize with the other child, recognize the difficulty she faces dealing with your child, and respect her willingness to play with *and tolerate* your child. Be sure to praise the great qualities she brings to the friendship. If there is a fight, apologize to the friend's mother, make amends, and defuse the situation, as this parent describes: *"We try to talk to the kids about the problems and help them see what went wrong and what they could do next time. A lot of times we leave well enough alone, but if bad words are said or someone is made fun of, we step in and talk to all the kids. If our child needs time to calm down, then we have him go to his room for a few minutes."* You have to walk a very fine line of diplomacy, and it can be tough, but who said it was going to be a rose garden? But hang on, it is going to be all right! *Yes*, it is a rose garden, with lots of thorns.

Create Social Opportunities

Your child needs opportunities to practice the social skills you are teaching him, and, if he's like most bipolar children, you will have to go out of your way to create events, activities, and play dates in order to engage other children. These activities don't have to be elaborate or expensive. They can be as simple as:

• *Home activities:* Invite kids to come over to cook together, get involved in rock painting, or play board games. Make it attractive to spend time at your house by having sports equipment such as a basketball hoop. Even some video games are OK! Check with other parents or game shops to select games with safe themes, such as sports that your child enjoys.

• *Theme parties:* This is no different from what you would do with any child without bipolar disorder. For girls, sleepovers or theme parties can be a great event, including movies, board games, painting, crafts, makeup, braids, dress up, and music, just to name a few things. Boys also seem to like movies and sports (often a series). You could have a party around the Super Bowl or the playoffs of your child's favorite sport. "*I try to help my kids participate in 'trendy' things as much as is reasonable,"* said one mother. *"For example, when Pokemon cards were popular, I let them buy them so they would have something in common with other kids."* Just pick some ideas and get going!

• *Team sports:* Older kids can play ice hockey, lacrosse, soccer, track and field, or basketball; if your child is too rambunctious for contact sports, consider tennis or swimming. In fact, swimming is very rhythmic and relaxing for your bipolar child. It is individual activity that frees your child from having to get along *all* the time.

• *Clubs:* Structured programs such as Boy Scouts or Indian Guides can be a good social setting to explore many interests, especially if Dad is willing to participate. Take this up only if one of you is willing and able to do it—it is not worth pushing yourself to try to fit in too many activities. The secret is to pick and choose the ones that work for your family.

• *Pets:* Sometimes having an appealing pet can be a social icebreaker for a socially shy bipolar child. One family got their anxiety-prone son a dog and went into training with him to become a social therapy team. According to the mother, *"He often talks with her, gets his exercise by walking with her, and when with her if he meets people—she's a yellow lab who draws people to her—he feels comfortable enough to have small social conversations."*

As I mentioned in Chapter 8, sports can be a great way to break from the dull daily routine, as well as an important social opportunity for bipolar children. In my practice, I actually have six children who are ice hockey goalies! I don't know which is the chicken and which is the egg, so to speak, but it seems hard to contain these children without an outlet to allow them to let off steam. The speed and intensity of the game is a good channel for their energy, plus it helps them establish team friendship and gain a sense of belonging. Remember, as in everything else, practice moderation. Bipolar kids are very excitable, and once they get stuck in overdrive, it's hard to get them to reboot. Parents get hyped up too. Find low-key activities so your child won't be in adrenaline overdrive all the time. I've had parents ask for stimulants to help their bipolar child improve performance. Beware of getting so caught up in the pressure to perform that you forget the healthy reasons you got your child involved in a sport in the first place.

One other caution: be careful not to overdo it with outside activities. Two activities a week outside the home are more than anyone can cope

---

Tips for Successful Socializing

- Set up play dates.
- Reach out to parents to send their kids; you need your own social skills sharpened, too—it's a two-part deal!
- Choose friends they like (like we do as adults).
- Select children *and* parents who will cooperate.
- Prime the kids and plan for the play date.
- Supervise the kids discreetly.
- Pull them aside and give feedback.
- Give positive feedback whenever possible.
- Limit the time to a maximum of 1–2 hours.
- Utilize sports, scouting, and home activities as opportunities to bond.
- Limit out-of-home activities to two per week.
- Check out social skills support groups and programs.

---

with, given schoolwork and doctor's appointments! Even families who don't have special needs children could benefit from drawing the line at being involved in too many activities. Your child can succeed academically as well, so don't look to sports scholarships as the only gateway to success in life for your bipolar child.

Investigate whether your child's school offers social skills groups, lunch buddies, or other activities for kids who are challenged socially. Community mental health centers or clinicians also may offer social skills groups.

Helping Your Child Handle Rejection

Rejection is inevitable for all of us. When something goes wrong with your child's relationships, you may even identify and feel rejected yourself. The first rule is to disengage yourself emotionally so you can be a strong anchor for your child. Try to empathize without identifying with your child—feeling miserable yourself will not help your child learn to be resilient.

The second rule is to *teach*, or, rather, *influence* (as you model) how human chemistry works. Some people are not a good match with others. While we all want to be liked and accepted, there are times that things don't work out. Sometimes children will abandon, ignore, or exclude your child, and it will break your heart. They might suddenly pick a different table in the lunchroom. Teach your child not to mope, feel sorry for herself, think less of herself, or pine for the other children's approval or acceptance. Teach her that it is healthy to let go and that new doors will open. She will feel better, gain self-respect, and make more friends in the long run. *"I do coach her on friendships,"* said one mother about her daughter. *"I encourage her to smile, even when she doesn't feel like it. I encourage her to be kind to everyone. She is very good at this, because she is truly compassionate and empathetic."*

Sometimes it makes sense to let go of a relationship that is tough. Help your child identify over time if this is the situation. You can figure it out from what your child tells you. He may tell you about how other children don't include him or describe the lunchroom scene: Who sits with whom? How do the children decide who to sit with? You already know who is popular and who your child wants to be with, but try to identify possible friends who are solid, genuine, caring, and talented. Nurture clear and healthy thinking in your child about choosing the right friends. You can't control this too much, because he has to work a lot of this out on his own, but he can benefit from your dispassionate input. Teach your child to roll with the punches, move on, and look for people who love him. Show him how as adults we learn to respect and treasure our relationships with those who appreciate us without pandering to the perceived elite. My friend, it's not worth it for you, and it's not worth it for your child, either! Validate his feelings and tell your child, "don't try too hard."

On the other hand, not all feedback from other children is a sign of rejection. The reality is that your child has to have friends and they are going to give her feedback. It will be raw, direct, and to the point: "You are being a jerk" or "I'm not listening to you. Why does it always have to be your way? I am out of here!" When this happens, it is easy to get upset with your child or feel helpless. But to a degree, it is important for your child to get this kind of feedback. When you correct her behavior, she will see it as criticism. Although you are trying to teach her the same thing as her friends, there comes a time when it is seen as too much criticism. It is really better if she hears it from friends and in reasonable doses. Remember that corrective feedback and a tolerable amount of "justifiable" outbursts do not equal outright rejection. Let your child process the information and let her grow through the feedback. One mom gives her daughter opportunities to process difficult experiences and mend fences, if neces-

---

Tips for Handling Rejection of Your Child

- Disengage emotionally.
- Empathize but don't identify.
- Teach resilient thinking.
- Let go of very difficult relationships.
- Teach your child not to try too hard.
- Let your child process valid feedback from peers.

---

sary, by taking responsibility for her actions: *"I remind her that her behaviors sometimes have a lot to do with how others respond to her."* You do not have to intervene every single time—practice occasional "masterly inactivity." In addition, bipolar children can also go through phases, falling in and out of favor with different children. Try to take it all in stride.

Rejection by peers and inability to relate to children his own age can lead to your child's hanging out with the "wrong crowd"—children who are substantially younger or older or who use substances, smoke, are truant, and generally get in trouble may seem less threatening for a child who feels like a misfit himself. *"It's as though, since he does not believe he is good enough, he'll hang with others who are worse off than him."* For this reason, close monitoring of your child's social connections is essential, especially as he approaches high school when the temptation to get involved in risky behaviors can increase for all children.

Getting Along at School

School is usually a child's most significant social arena, as children spend most of their day there, so it is a critical factor in developing self-esteem and social skills. One of the biggest problems parents report their child having at school is finding friends and dealing with peers. This can be intensified if your child spends much of her time in special classes, programs, or schools.

There are a number of ways to help your child find friends at school. One way is to hang out at the door while picking up your child from school to see whom your child gravitates toward and get to know other parents. You could even ask the teacher's opinion on who might make a good match for your child. Once you identify suitable children who your child likes with cooperative parents, you can start setting up play dates.

For many children, extracurricular activities provide a structured social environment as well as an opportunity to be good at something besides academics. Teachers and other staff can also help ensure that the bipolar child isn't isolated by setting up a buddy system or making sure that the child has someone to sit with on field trips and in the lunchroom.

Unfortunately, schools are rife with social hazards for children with bipolar disorder, who may appear different and vulnerable to other kids—what some researchers call the "provocative victim." They are prone to bullying and harassment and, because of their volatile natures, respond with aggressive behavior, earning themselves detention or suspension. This can go on over many years, leading to a troubled and less-than-desirable image among peers and their parents. How can we address this critical problem when we seem to have used up all of the school administration and faculty's goodwill just getting help with your child's academic needs?

So what do you do when . . .

• *Your child comes home upset because he's constantly teased and yet the teacher supposedly does nothing about it?* The best long-term solution is to introduce an anti-bullying program to your school. Do some Internet research to find program materials available that train teachers and students to identify antisocial behavior and address it. You may want to share this idea with the school, but remember to approach this sensitively, involving one or two key people at the school who are receptive to the idea. Don't just go to the teachers and start telling them what to do. In the meantime, you might raise the issue with the principal, asking to speak with him in confidence if it seems appropriate (you don't want the principal or the teacher saying something to your child) and asking for input on what he thinks is going on. Remember, you have only your child's version of the story. If the complete story suggests that the teacher is ignoring bullying, you might ask for the principal's assistance in addressing the problem and offer to help in any way you can. Principals are pretty sensitive to this stuff, as school systems often feel liable if they know about a problem and do nothing to address it. Follow up your conversation with a thank-you note. If the problem continues, speak to the principal again and again offer your assistance. See if other parents share your concern (some certainly do), and make it an issue for the PTA to raise.

- *You get calls from parents saying your child is bullying the other kids at recess?* This happens too, of course. Is your child being fully and appropriately treated? Is your therapist offering concrete suggestions for dealing with the problem? Bullying is quite a responsive target for behavior therapies, but it may require a professional's assistance. Don't attack the problem by yourself if things are not working. Also, explore whether your child's medication, if any, is adjusted adequately to reduce aggressive behavior.

If the situation is dire—for instance, if your child is a danger to himself or others—and no interventions seem to make a difference, it might be necessary to change schools or find a different setting, such as a therapeutic school or residential treatment center (RTC), that can better meet your child's needs. See Chapter 9 for additional discussion about when to pursue this option.

Bonding with Other Adults

Relationships with other adults in your child's life can give him the additional support and encouragement he needs. You get to be the same old mom or dad, but other role models—aunts and uncles, cousins, neighbors, friends, and other adults such as counselors or coaches—can give your child a new perspective and help look out for her at school and in the neighborhood. Some of these relationships may arise naturally through play dates or extracurricular activities. These are the people who will appear on your child's "support tree."

One parent found other parents who were willing to help: "*My daughter really wants to be liked and is quite kind to her friends. She has met a couple of very nice girls whose mothers have taken a liking to her. I have shared some of her difficulties with these mothers without actually naming her disorder. They have become coaches for her, and she has had several successful sleepovers because of this.*" By building relationships with other parents, you have a better opportunity to work behind the scenes to coach, intervene, and orchestrate peer activities.

Talking with the other significant adults in your child's life on special occasions, such as holidays, can create natural opportunities for them to bond and let your kid lap up the luxury of the extended support. For example, you can prepare a kind aunt to look out for your child. Tell the aunt that your child really loves her hugs and talks about how kind she is or how elegant she looks—the list is endless if you look for positive links between a relative and your child. Catch those vibes and transmit them back to the child and the relative and let them continue to nurture that positive link. Teach your child to address them with their names—"Aunt Mary, how are you?"—when they call instead of saying just "Hi" when Aunt Mary is trying to be nice. Your job is to facilitate and cultivate a positive network of caring adults to support your child.

On the other hand, some adults can be intrusive helpers who may not be all that helpful but only too eager to offer unwelcome advice ("There's nothing wrong with this child") or antagonize you in other ways. These people come in two types: those who do not care about your family but are happy enough to dish out free advice and those who care about you but are narrow-minded or have antiquated ideas about mental illness and child rearing. With the first type, ignore them and don't waste your time trying to set them straight. With the second type, try to keep an open mind and educate them about your child's disorder. Again, put on your manager's hat and gently steer your child away from this influence. Either way, don't get defensive or lose your temper. You know what your child needs.

Looking Ahead

Home, school, and the social arena are the domains in which our children spend their days, and I hope the chapters in Part III have given you a lot of good ideas for adopting the RAINBOW principles to boost your bipolar child's happiness in the world. These principles will serve you well as your child grows and changes in the years ahead.

A Final Word

What can you look forward to as your son or daughter navigates the rest of childhood and enters the uncharted territory of adolescence and adulthood? I firmly believe that once your child's moods have been stabilized and you and your family have learned to use the RAINBOW principles, you can look forward to a brighter future. You and your child can survive the crises, the challenges, and the changes that will come your way, and your child can grow up to be a healthy, functional adult. What I want to leave you with more than anything else as a final offering is hope.

We don't know from the current research whether bipolar children grow up to develop the adult form of bipolar disorder, continue to have the pediatric variant, or substantially recover. Some research indicates that many do develop a cycling and persistent form of the adult variant. Whatever the predictions may be, you can remain centered on working toward recovery. Our goal in treatment is to strive for that precious recovery, tracking the symptoms and striving for long-term stability. You now have at your disposal a lot of the tools that we use in our clinic to reach that rainbow.

In my experience, children do particularly well if they have two things in their favor: intelligence and strong family support with skilled, compassionate parenting. The former is mostly endowed at birth; you generally don't wrack your brain over these but simply enjoy the way your child was delivered to you. You've already shown your dedication to and support of your child, as well as your motivation to become an even more skilled parent than you were. The more you model skills with your child, the more you pass them on so your child will be able to handle bipolar dis-

order with aplomb and resilience as he or she grows and matures. You're
providing your child with important skills that will last a lifetime.

Onward and Upward

Meanwhile, you'll continue to have good days and not-so-good days.
Sometimes your day-to-day coping strategies will be taxed to the max.
Measured optimism and the ability to let go of the need to control the situation can help you weather the storm. Your doctor should be able to provide additional advice for coping and reassure you that things will
improve with time. Here are some additional tips for making it through
these toughest of times and coming out the other side intact and whole.

Make Lifestyle Changes

Often parents make changes to their lives in order to make things work
better for their bipolar child and themselves. This can include changing
jobs, having one parent stay home from work, working part-time, maintaining flexible shifts, or even starting a home-based business to be more
available to help with homework, doctors' appointments, and other
demands. One family I know moved to be closer to an appropriate school
and healthcare providers. This may not be the ultimate solution, but it
does open up possibilities for how you might take some of the pressure off
and make it easier for everyone to cope in particularly difficult circumstances.

Seek Therapy

What I find often is that parents do poorly if things get overwhelming and
they themselves are just not coping. You may resist seeing someone for
therapy, but getting a smart and caring therapist will help you navigate
your life better. I am not talking about you participating in RAINBOW
therapy, but just therapy for yourself as an individual. Work with your
therapist to find tangible solutions to help you weather the storm. Your
therapist should also be able to provide wisdom, perspective, and strength
at times when you need solace. A spouse or best friend who serves as your
"rock" may crumble if leaned on too hard and too long.

Be Open to New Opinions

Don't be afraid to talk to other professionals when you feel caught in a conundrum. Getting a new opinion from another doctor, therapist, or other clinician may offer a fresh perspective, along with new tools and techniques that may work. Sometimes, when families seek another opinion, especially when the first doctor collaborates with the second one, a better treatment plan emerges.

Step Back and Reevaluate

If you have tried a host of options for getting through a particularly rough patch and things are still not making sense, what's going on? Could you or your spouse be depressed or suffering from some other problem that a doctor could help with? Could your child be dealing with something other than bipolar illness, such as stress over the death of a family member or pet, tests coming up, friends moving away, parents fighting, Dad losing a job, or Mom having been diagnosed with a major illness? Sometimes waiting out the tough times for a little while will help you figure out what is happening in the context of your child's and your current state of health and the stress level in the environment your family lives in, allowing you to determine the best course of action. If symptoms begin to return or a pattern resumes, it may be time to act.

Connect with Other Parents

Remember, all of your needs cannot be met at home, and you need other places to recharge your batteries. Do you have one or more friends you can relate to and confide in? If not, it's time to make these connections, whether at work, at church/temple/mosque, at the day care center, or somewhere else. Many parents seek—and get—guidance and hope from other parents. Support groups such as CABF can be a great resource for parents in crisis, and the chat rooms on their websites are a place to share your feelings and find understanding. Other parents are often the best source of hope because they have traveled the same path and found success. In the box on the next page are some insights about what made the biggest difference in the lives of other parents dealing with bipolar disorder.

What's the One Piece of Advice Other Parents Offer?

We asked members of CABF to share their stories with us and offer bits of wisdom based on their experience for coping with the demands of bipolar disorder. Here are the kinds of things they told us:

"Find a support group. Other parents are the only ones who will take you seriously when you say that your 6-year-old has been trying to commit suicide. Other people think that you are exaggerating. Other parents can help you to find the doctors who are willing and able to provide real help."

"Seek the best medical advice, a doctor who specializes in the disease, and surround yourself with a support system of therapists, doctors, etc."

"Understand and accept the illness ASAP and what it means to your child, your family, and your relationships within. Also, as hard and painful as it can be, have the courage to do the right thing."

"Try to get the total support of your spouse, be a team together, and don't work against each other."

"Accurate information helps. If you meet with success in treatment, keep in mind that relapses are probably in store so as to avoid devastation."

"Surround yourself with supportive and understanding friends and get rid of those who are not."

"Write a letter to the principal, teacher, and superintendent for special certified education services!!! Get it done."

"Never give up! No matter how much work it seems to be. When parents give up hope, they quit trying. Then their children lose hope, and worse things happen."

"Fight for your child; don't let the doctors and family and friends think you are making something out of nothing. Look for information and be your child's advocate."

"Talk to other parents, find the best medical care from parent references, and find a doctor who is accessible. Get emotional support and medical support. Remember that your child is important and needs your attention. Also talk with your other children and explain the illness."

More information and support groups can be found at *www.bpkids.org*.

Appendices

Principles for Meeting the Challenge of Bipolar Disorder

Keeping the following principles in mind will help you cope with the day-to-day challenges of bipolar disorder. Post them on the refrigerator or copy them onto note cards and keep them as a handy reference for stressful occasions. Anchor yourself with these thoughts along your life journey. Think of life as a train ride that you learn to appreciate for all that you experience in each moment, rather than focusing on the destination as a goal.

1. **Get educated.** Understanding what's going on can help you stay calm, manage your fears, and deal more effectively with problems.
2. **Be realistic.** Appreciate your child as he is and don't expect miracles of your child or yourself. Good things will still happen!
3. **Everything in moderation.** Don't stress yourself in the quest for perfection. Do your best with what's important in moderation and let some things slide.
4. **Be flexible.** Unpredictability is the norm with bipolar disorder. Being flexible and resilient is a matter of survival.
5. **Have fun and play.** Make opportunities to play, relax, and participate in the things that make life worth living. Look after yourself. Reboot the strategies for doing so from time to time! Don't take yourself too seriously, and look for the joy in life.
6. **Keep your sense of humor.** You can find plenty of humor if you keep things in perspective. Even if you are not funny, identify and surround yourself with supportive people who can offer strength and stimulate laughter.
7. **Stay compassionate.** Try to remain compassionate and loving even when your child is at her worst. Try to remember that, as hard as it is for you, it's even harder for your son or daughter.
8. **Make connections.** Isolation is likely to intensify your stress and unhappiness. Build a support network through your church, school, other community institutions, and nonprofit groups.

Child Mania Rating Scale—Parent Version (CMRS-P)

_____   _____   _____
Child's name   Date of birth   Case # / ID #
                         (mm/dd/yy)

Instructions

The following questions concern your child's mood and behavior in the **past month**. Please place a check mark or an × in a box for each item. Please consider it a problem if it is **causing trouble** and is beyond what is normal for your child's age. Check "Never/rarely" if the behavior is not causing trouble.

Does your child . . .	Never/ rarely	Some- times	Often	Very often
1. Have periods of feeling super-happy for hours or days at a time and being extremely wound up and excited, such as feeling "on top of the world"?	0	1	2	3
2. Feel irritable, cranky, or mad for hours or days at a time?	0	1	2	3
3. Think that he or she can be anything or do anything (e.g., leader, best basketball player, rapper, millionaire, princess) beyond what is usual for that age?	0	1	2	3
4. Believe that he or she has unrealistic abilities or powers that are unusual, and may try to act upon them, which causes trouble?	0	1	2	3
5. Need less sleep than usual yet does not feel tired the next day?	0	1	2	3
6. Have periods of too much energy?	0	1	2	3

_____

Does your child . . .	Never/ rarely	Some- times	Often	Very often
7. Have periods when he or she talks too much, too loud, or a mile a minute?	0	1	2	3
8. Have periods of racing thoughts that his or her mind cannot slow down (it seems that your child's mouth cannot keep up with his or her mind)?	0	1	2	3
9. Talk so fast that he or she jumps from topic to topic?	0	1	2	3
10. Rush around doing things nonstop?	0	1	2	3
11. Have trouble staying on track and is easily drawn to what is happening around him or her?	0	1	2	3
12. Do many more things than usual or is unusually productive or highly creative?	0	1	2	3
13. Behave in a sexually inappropriate way (e.g., talks dirty, exposes him- or herself, plays with private parts, masturbates, makes sex phone calls, humps on dogs, plays sex games, touches others sexually)?	0	1	2	3
14. Go and talk to strangers inappropriately or is more socially outgoing than usual?	0	1	2	3
15. Do things that are unusual for him or her that are foolish or risky (e.g., jumping off heights, ordering CDs with your credit cards, giving things away)?	0	1	2	3
16. Have rage attacks or intense and prolonged temper tantrums?	0	1	2	3
17. Crack jokes or pun more than usual, laugh loud, or act silly in a way that is out of the ordinary?	0	1	2	3
18. Experience rapid mood swings?	0	1	2	3
19. Have any suspicious or strange thoughts?	0	1	2	3
20. Hear voices that nobody else can hear?	0	1	2	3
21. See things that nobody else can see?	0	1	2	3

Please send comments to: Mpavuluri@psych.uic.edu

Child Mania Rating Scale—Teacher Version (CMRS-T)

Child's name	Date of birth (mm/dd/yy)	Case # / ID #

Instructions

The following questions concern the child's mood and behavior. Please place a check mark or an × in a box for each item. Please consider it a problem if it is causing trouble and is beyond what is normal for the child's age. Check "Never/rarely" if the behavior is not causing trouble.

Does the child . . .	Never/ rarely	Some- times	Often	Very often
1. Have periods of feeling super-happy for hours or days at a time and being extremely wound up and excited, such as feeling "on top of the world"?	0	1	2	3
2. Feel irritable, cranky, or mad for hours or days at a time?	0	1	2	3
3. Think that he or she can be anything or do anything (e.g., leader, best basketball player, rapper, millionaire, princess) beyond what is usual for that age?	0	1	2	3
4. Believe that he or she has unrealistic abilities or powers that are unusual, and may try to act upon them, which causes trouble?	0	1	2	3
5. Have periods of too much energy?	0	1	2	3

Does the child . . .	Never/ rarely	Some-times	Often	Very often
6. Have periods when he or she talks too much, too loud, or a mile a minute?	0	1	2	3
7. Have periods of racing thoughts that his or her mind cannot slow down (it seems that the child's mouth cannot keep up with his or her mind)?	0	1	2	3
8. Talk so fast that he or she jumps from topic to topic?	0	1	2	3
9. Rush around doing things nonstop?	0	1	2	3
10. Have trouble staying on track and is easily drawn to what is happening around him or her?	0	1	2	3
11. Do many more things than usual or is unusually productive or highly creative?	0	1	2	3
12. Behave in a sexually inappropriate way (e.g., talks dirty, exposes him- or herself, plays with private parts, masturbates, makes sex phone calls, humps on dogs, plays sex games, touches others sexually)?	0	1	2	3
13. Go and talk to strangers inappropriately or is more socially outgoing than usual?	0	1	2	3
14. Do things that are unusual for him or her that are foolish or risky (e.g., jumping off heights, giving things away)?	0	1	2	3
15. Have rage attacks or intense and prolonged temper tantrums?	0	1	2	3
16. Crack jokes or pun more than usual, laugh loud, or act silly in a way that is out of the ordinary?	0	1	2	3
17. Experience rapid mood swings?	0	1	2	3
18. Have any suspicious or strange thoughts?	0	1	2	3
19. Hear voices that nobody else can hear?	0	1	2	3
20. See things that nobody else can see?	0	1	2	3

Please send comments to: Mpavuluri@psych.uic.edu

Medication: Tracking the History of Response

Name: _____

Medication + dose	Response CGI score Worse Better	Side effects/reason for discontinuation
methylphenidate/Ritalin, Concerta, etc.	−3 −2 −1 0 +1 +2 +3	_____
dextroamphetamine/Dexedrine	−3 −2 −1 0 +1 +2 +3	_____
other stimulants:	−3 −2 −1 0 +1 +2 +3	_____
atomoxetine/Strattera	−3 −2 −1 0 +1 +2 +3	_____
imipramine/Tofranil	−3 −2 −1 0 +1 +2 +3	_____
clonidine/Catapres	−3 −2 −1 0 +1 +2 +3	_____
guanfacine/Tenex	−3 −2 −1 0 +1 +2 +3	_____
mixed salts/Adderall XR, etc.	−3 −2 −1 0 +1 +2 +3	_____
other ADHD Rx:	−3 −2 −1 0 +1 +2 +3	_____
lithium	−3 −2 −1 0 +1 +2 +3	_____
divalproex/Depakote	−3 −2 −1 0 +1 +2 +3	_____
lamotrigine/Lamictal	−3 −2 −1 0 +1 +2 +3	_____
carbamazepine/Tegretol	−3 −2 −1 0 +1 +2 +3	_____
oxcarbazepine/Trileptal	−3 −2 −1 0 +1 +2 +3	_____
topiramate/Topamax	−3 −2 −1 0 +1 +2 +3	_____
gabapentin/Neurontin	−3 −2 −1 0 +1 +2 +3	_____
tiagabine/Gabitril	−3 −2 −1 0 +1 +2 +3	_____
zonisamide/Zonegran	−3 −2 −1 0 +1 +2 +3	_____

Medication + dose	Response CGI score Worse	Better	Side effects/reason for discontinuation
chlorpromazine/Thorazine	−3 −2 −1 0 +1 +2 +3		_____
haloperidol/Haldol	−3 −2 −1 0 +1 +2 +3		_____
other neuroleptic:	−3 −2 −1 0 +1 +2 +3		_____
risperidone/Risperdal	−3 −2 −1 0 +1 +2 +3		_____
paliperidone/Invega	−3 −2 −1 0 +1 +2 +3		_____
olanzapine/Zyprexa	−3 −2 −1 0 +1 +2 +3		_____
clozapine/Clozaril	−3 −2 −1 0 +1 +2 +3		_____
quetiapine/Seroquel	−3 −2 −1 0 +1 +2 +3		_____
ziprasidone/Geodon	−3 −2 −1 0 +1 +2 +3		_____
aripiprazole/Abilify	−3 −2 −1 0 +1 +2 +3		_____
olanzapine + fluoxetine/Symbyax	−3 −2 −1 0 +1 +2 +3		_____
fluvoxamine/Luvox	−3 −2 −1 0 +1 +2 +3		_____
escitalopram/Lexapro	−3 −2 −1 0 +1 +2 +3		_____
venlafaxine/Effexor	−3 −2 −1 0 +1 +2 +3		_____
trazodone/Desyrel	−3 −2 −1 0 +1 +2 +3		_____
fluoxetine/Prozac	−3 −2 −1 0 +1 +2 +3		_____
paroxetine/Paxil	−3 −2 −1 0 +1 +2 +3		_____
sertraline/Zoloft	−3 −2 −1 0 +1 +2 +3		_____
citalopram/Celexa	−3 −2 −1 0 +1 +2 +3		_____
clomipramine/Anafranil	−3 −2 −1 0 +1 +2 +3		_____
bupropion/Wellbutrin	−3 −2 −1 0 +1 +2 +3		_____
duloxetine/Cymbalta	−3 −2 −1 0 +1 +2 +3		_____
benzodiazepines/Ativan, Xanax, Klonopin, etc.	−3 −2 −1 0 +1 +2 +3		_____
Other antidepressant	−3 −2 −1 0 +1 +2 +3		_____
Other medication	−3 −2 −1 0 +1 +2 +3		_____
Other medication	−3 −2 −1 0 +1 +2 +3		_____

Pediatric Side Effects Checklist (P-SEC)

This checklist is to be completed by parent, child, or patient. This will help identify the adverse effects of the medication(s). Please read through the list and check (✓) in the appropriate box.

Patient name: _____ ID: _____ Date: _____

Problems	None	Mild/ sometimes but tolerable	Moderate/ interferes somewhat	Severe/ interferes a lot
Gastrointestinal system				
Discomfort in the stomach				
Constipation				
Diarrhea				
Increased appetite				
Decreased appetite				
Nausea/vomiting				
Central nervous system				
Muscle trembling/shaking				
Sleepiness				
Difficulty falling asleep				
Muscle stiffness				
Stiff jaw				
Problems concentrating				
Problems with memory				
Restlessness/wanting to pace				
Irritation/agitation				

This checklist accounts for most of the possible side effects seen with medications utilized in psychopharmacotherapy.

From *What Works for Bipolar Kids* by Mani Pavuluri. Copyright 2008 by The Guilford Press.

Problems	None	Mild/ sometimes but tolerable	Moderate/ interferes somewhat	Severe/ interferes a lot
Problems with speech				
Dizziness/lightheadedness				
Headache				
Seizures				
Nightmares/vivid dreams				
Blurring of vision				
Excessive drooling				
Increased sweating				
Increased thirst				
Dry mouth/eyes				
Endocrine system				
Feeling cold/hot				
Weight gain				
Weight loss				
Fatigue/tiredness				
Breast cyst				
Changes in menstrual periods				
Mood/behavior changes				
Depression/feeling sad				
Excitability				
Feeling anxious				
Aggression				
Panic attacks				
Cardiovascular system				
Palpitations				
Blackouts/loss of consciousness				
Chest pain				
Immune system				
Frequent infections				

Problems	None	Mild/ sometimes but tolerable	Moderate/ interferes somewhat	Severe/ interferes a lot
Skin				
Rash				
Acne				
Hair loss				
Renal system				
Increased urination				
Bed wetting				
Frothy urine/red urine				
Sexual concerns/problems				
Sexual concerns/problems				
Other				
Allergic reaction				
Other, please specify:				

Please indicate your current medications here.

Medication	Dose

Medications Used for Bipolar Disorder in Children

In the following lists the generic name of each psychopharmacological agent is followed by the trade (brand) name.

First-generation antipsychotics
Chlorpromazine: Thorazine
Fluphenazine: Prolixin
Haloperidol: Haldol
Loxapine: Loxitane
Mesoridazine: Serentil
Molindone: Moban
Perphenazine: Trilafon
Pimozide: Orap
Trifluoperazine: Stelazine
Thioridazine: Mellaril
Thiothixene: Navane

Second-generation antipsychotics
Aripiprazole: Abilify
Clozapine: Clozaril; generic clozapine
Olanzapine: Zyprexa
Paliperidone: Invega
Quetiapine: Seroquel
Risperidone: Risperdal; Risperdal Consta
Ziprasidone: Geodon

First-generation antidepressants
Heterocyclics
Amitriptyline: Elavil

CR, controlled release; ER or XR, extended release; SR, sustained release; CD, controlled delivery; LA, long-acting formulation.

From *What Works for Bipolar Kids* by Mani Pavuluri. Copyright 2008 by The Guilford Press.

Imipramine: Tofranil
Clomipramine: Anafranil
Desipramine: Norpramin
Doxepin: Sinequan
Maprotiline: Ludiomil
Nortriptyline: Pamelor
Protriptyline: Vivactil
Trimipramine: Surmontil

Dibenzoxazepine
Amoxapine: Asendin

Phenylpiperazine
Trazodone: Desyrel; generic trazodone; Trazolan

Monoamine oxidase inhibitors
Phenelzine: Nardil
Selegiline: Emsam
Tranylcypromine: Parnate

Second-generation antidepressants
Fluoxetine: Prozac
Sertraline: Zoloft
Paroxetine: Paxil; Paxil CR; generic paroxetine
Fluvoxamine: Luvox
Citalopram: Celexa
Escitalopram: Lexapro
Venlafaxine: Effexor
Nefazodone: Serzone
Mirtazapine: Remeron
Bupropion: Wellbutrin; Zyban
Duloxetine: Cymbalta

Mood stabilizers
Lithium: Eskalith; Eskalith CR; Lithobid SR; lithium citrate; lithium carbonate
Valproate: Depacon; Depakote; Depakene
Lamotrigine: Lamictal
Carbamazepine: Tegretol
Oxcarbazepine: Trileptal
Gabapentin: Neurontin

Tiagabine: Gabitril
Topiramate: Topamax
Zonisamide: Zonegran

Anxiolytics/sedative–hypnotics
Benzodiazepines
Diazepam: Valium
Lorazepam: Ativan
Clonazepam: Klonopin
Alprazolam: Xanax
Oxazepam: Serax
Temazepam: Restoril
Midazolam: Versed

Buspirone: BuSpar
Pregabalin: Lyrica
Zolpidem: Ambien
Zaleplon: Sonata
Eszopiclone: Lunesta
Ramelteon: Rozerem

Adjuvant medications
Clonidine: Catapres
Guanfacine: Tenex

Psychostimulants
Methylphenidate: Ritalin; Ritalin LA; Ritalin SR; Concerta; Daytrana; Metadate
    ER; Metadate CD; Methylin; Cylert
Dexmethylphenidate: Focalin; FocalinXR
Dextroamphetamine: Dexedrine; Dextrostat
Mixed amphetamine salts (Adderall; Adderall XR)
Modafinil: Provigil
Atomoxetine: Strattera; generic Attentin

Miscellaneous medications
Propranolol: Inderal
Desmopressin: DDAVP

Daily Mood Calendar

Name _____ Month _____

Color in the square using a color that best describes your overall mood for each part of the day.

Key:

Blue = Sad
Red = Angry/explosive
Gray = Crabby/irritable
Yellow = Happy
Orange = Silly
Green = Neutral/fair
Purple = Worried

Week 1   Date _____ To _____

	Sunday	Monday	Tuesday	Wednesday	Thursday	Friday	Saturday
Morning							
Afternoon							
Evening							

Week 2   Date _____ To _____

	Sunday	Monday	Tuesday	Wednesday	Thursday	Friday	Saturday
Morning							
Afternoon							
Evening							

Framework
for a Physician–School Teleconference

1. Assess individual education needs for the child.
2. Determine an appropriate educational plan.
3. Learn about bipolar disorder.
4. Address handling emotional issues at school.
5. Discuss learning problems and academic difficulties.
6. Discuss additional services such as occupational therapy, speech therapy, and social skills training.
7. Discuss communication between family and school.
8. Discuss medication issues.

Usually the teleconference is conducted with the special education director, the school principal, social worker, class teachers, resource teachers, the family, and any additional professionals involved in the child's school setting. The psychiatrist/clinician should be available on speakerphone to participate in this school conference. This service is usually not covered by private insurance and is typically billed as self-pay.

    1. **Assess needs.** Although most children with bipolar disorder typically have the same sorts of problems at school, each child is unique in his or her struggles in the school environment. As a part of our conference, information is gathered from parents, the school team, and the clinician to determine areas of strength and weakness. These are then the foundation for planning appropriate school interventions.

    2. **Determine an appropriate educational plan.** The team will determine the appropriate educational plan according to the needs assessment.

    This plan may include:

    a. classroom interventions and assistance
    b. a 504 plan
    c. an IEP
    d. an IEP with a classroom aide
    e. therapeutic school
    f. residential placement

Recommendations and discussion of the specific aspects of the plan will occur within the team.

3. **Learn about bipolar disorder.** Bipolar disorder is complicated and affects the child in multiple ways. The nature of bipolar disorder and how it presents in the particular child is carefully described to school personnel and shared with parents so that everyone is in agreement as what to expect with the child in the classroom and in settings such as the lunchroom, gym class, and so forth. The school team needs to understand the chronic and cyclical nature of the illness and how that may affect the child's learning. Potential risks, how the illness impacts relationships, and self-esteem are also discussed, so that a sense of empathy can be established between the child and his or her school team.

4. **Address handling emotional issues at school.**

- Suggestions are given to the school team (social worker, teacher) so that they may take the lead on ensuring that services are provided throughout the school year.
- The RAINBOW program is introduced to the school team (social worker, teacher) who will be conducting individual sessions at school.
- The team is encouraged to give the child additional leadership responsibilities for a specific task such as taking attendance sheets to the office, keeping the calendar, or cleaning the blackboard.
- The buddy system is encouraged to help the child with social relationships. For instance, the child can be seated next to a person who is likely to interact with this child. This will encourage developing friendships and shared time in the lunchroom rather than designating a specific buddy and asking that buddy to play with this child.
- It is expected that the child will receive one-to-one sessions in addition to pep talks given by the class resource teacher.
- The pep talks can be anywhere between 10 and 15 minutes, one to seven times a week, based on the need.

5. **Discuss learning problems and academic difficulties.** Depending on the child's learning difficulties, services are set up in or out of the classroom so that

the child is able to learn effectively without feeling ostracized. Problems such as inability to concentrate will be handled through medications, and the school team will be encouraged to provide information for medical visits so that concentration can be monitored effectively. The school team is encouraged to nurture areas of academic strength and to cultivate them so that the child has areas of accomplishment.

6. **Discuss additional services such as occupational therapy, speech therapy, and social skills training.** Social skills training, occupational therapy, and speech services need to be provided through the IEP. A discussion of these needs and their significance for the child will be highlighted.

7. **Discuss communication between family and school.** Communication with the family is encouraged. Parents are encouraged to talk with the child's teachers, and the teachers are encouraged to provide frequent notes, calls, and contact with the family. Teachers and parents are encouraged to give positive feedback not only to the child but also to each other about the techniques that the other party is implementing, in order to make the collaboration effective and synergistic.

8. **Discuss medication issues.** Medications being given to the child are described in detail along with side effects. The family is encouraged to notify the school when significant medication changes are made.

The philosophy of managing the child at school is based on making school a secure and safe environment, by building on the strengths of the child rather than dissecting behaviors and approaching each minor problem as a major obstacle. School staff often tell us that they have already tried most of the above strategies, or they raise problems such as the child not wanting to attend the classroom or being defiant or stubborn. Often it is critical to use these times as learning moments, and to use problem-solving strategies that would rescue the child out of these difficult situations. Working at problems collaboratively, involving the child, and giving choices within reason can help the child to help him- or herself. When the child remains stuck in making things difficult at school, he or she needs to be gently guided toward effective and constructive actions rather than affective and destructive ones. Forcing a difficult child to cooperate can increase the intensity of a situation and cause the child to fight back. Bipolar children typically respond better in a more collaborative fashion, discussing things before a crisis develops and avoiding struggles of power.

Resources

My Book Club for All Parents and Caregivers

The Parent's Tao Te Ching: Ancient Advice for Modern Parents, by William Martin (New York: Marlowe, 1999).—Underscores loving parent–child relationships—responding without judgment, emulating natural processes, and balancing doing and being.

Whale Done!: The Power of Positive Relationships, by Ken Blanchard (New York: Free Press, 2002).—Invaluable in managing the killer-whale–type rage in bipolar children by taming them with mutual trust.

Good Friends Are Hard to Find: Help Your Child Find, Make, and Keep Friends, by Fred Frankel (London: Perspective Publishing, 1996).—This is a great book that clearly lays out the details on how to learn to be a good friend and keep good friendships, especially emphasizing the role of parental supervision.

The Blessing of a Skinned Knee: Using Jewish Teachings to Raise Self-Reliant Children, by Wendy Mogel (Darby, PA: Diane, 2003).—Keeps trajectory of child development, hardships, pains, and gains of parenting in perspective.

Handbook of Psychopharmacotherapy: A Life-Span Approach, 2nd ed., by Mani Pavuluri and Philip Janicak (Philadelphia: Lippincott, Williams & Wilkins, 2007).—Gives a quick and comprehensive overview of the pharmacotherapy repertoire you need to know for your bipolar child or any patient with any psychiatric disorder, from pediatrics to geriatrics.

The Secret, by Rhonda Byrne (New York: Atria, 2006).—It gives away the secret of positive thinking and the law of attraction that says, "Like attracts like, so when you think a thought, you are also attracting like thoughts," just like a magnet.

Family Wisdom from the Monk Who Sold His Ferrari, by Robin Sharma (Carlsbad, CA: Hay House, 2003).—This book gives you insights into creating a family culture that is rich and enduring and brings balance to your lifestyle, allowing you to celebrate life with contentment and simplicity.

How to Talk So Kids Will Listen and Listen So Kids Will Talk, by Adele Faber and Elaine Mazlish (London: Piccadilly Press, 2001).—This book lays a foundation to bring about cooperation in the family, especially with children, and find alternatives to punishment and to yelling and screaming at home.

Recommended Websites

bpkids.org—The website of the Child and Adolescent Bipolar Foundation is a rich global resource for families and children with bipolar disorder, offering a great network in virtual space. It has a message board where you can get referrals and find out about support groups operating in your area or create your own support group. This will give you A–Z information in obtaining any relevant resources. *This is a must site to visit.*

bpchildresearch.org—This is the website of the Juvenile Bipolar Research Foundation, run by Janice Papolos and Demitri Papolos to encourage professional dialogue between clinical experts and interested clinicians. The Papoloses serve as great advocates for families with bipolar children.

nami.org—The special attractions of the National Alliance on Mental Illness (NAMI) are its families-to-families program and its visions-for-tomorrow program—a series of group tutorials from parent leaders to parents and caregivers of mentally ill children. You can graduate from their programs and go on to help others. They may have local branches in your region or allow you to connect to others.

dbsalliance.org—The Depression and Bipolar Support Alliance is a major organization for manic and depressive illnesses. CABF is linked as a sister organization.

bpchildren.com—Tracy Anglada operates a neat website, with the main attraction being the stories of those who experience the rollercoaster of bipolar disorder.

isbd.org—The website of the International Society for Bipolar Disorders contains links to a lot of scientific information on bipolar disorder, though not specifically about children. The society is a forum for researchers, clinicians, advocacy groups, and individuals dedicated to promoting international collaboration, education, research, and advances in treatment and other aspects of bipolar disorders.

blackdoginstitute.org.au—According to this Australian website, the Black Dog Institute is "an educational, research, clinical and community-oriented facility dedicated to improving understanding, diagnosis and treatment of mood disorders." Children are not a major focus, but the site contains a lot of information and links that parents may find useful.

bckidsmentalhealth.org—The F.O.R.C.E. (Families Organized for Recognition and Care Equality) Society for Kids Mental Health is a Canadian parents' organization based in British Columbia whose mission is "to promote and influence change in intervention and equality of care in children's mental health." The group operates skill-building seminars for parents, advocates for policy change, and offers links to helpful governmental information.

depression.mb.ca—The Mood Disorders Association of Manitoba is a self-help organization whose goal is "helping others to help themselves through peer support, education, and advocacy, promoting public awareness about mood disorders and empowering people to develop and manage mental wellness."

mooddisorderscanada.ca—The Mood Disorders Society of Canada provides links to a wealth of bipolar disorder resources in Canada and the United States.

youngminds.org.uk—Young Minds is a nonprofit organization in the United Kingdom dedicated to improving the mental health of all children and young people; it offers links to a lot of information on bipolar disorder.

Bibliography

Ambrosini, P. J. (2000). A review of pharmacotherapy of major depression in children and adolescents. *Psychiatric Services, 51,* 627–633.

Biederman, J., Faraone, S., Mick, E., et al. (1996). Attention-deficit/hyperactivity disorder and juvenile mania; an overlooked comorbidity? *Journal of the American Academy of Child and Adolescent Psychiatry, 35,* 997–1008.

Biederman, J., Mick, E., Spencer, T., et al. (2000). Therapeutic dilemmas in the pharmacotherapy of bipolar depression in the young. *Journal of Child and Adolescent Psychopharmacology, 10,* 185–192.

Carlson, G. A. (1990). Child and adolescent mania—diagnostic considerations. *Journal of Child Psychology and Psychiatry, 31,* 331–341.

Esposito-Smythers, C., Birmaher, B., Valeri, S., et al. (2006). Child comorbidity, maternal mood disorder, and perceptions of family functioning among bipolar youth. *Journal of the American Academy of Child and Adolescent Psychiatry, 45,* 955–964.

Faraone, S. V., Biederman, J., Mennin, D., et al. (1997). Attention-deficit/hyperactivity disorder with bipolar disorder: A familial subtype? *Journal of the American Academy of Child and Adolescent Psychiatry, 36,* 1378–1381.

Faraone, S. V., Biederman, J., Wozniak, J., et al. (1997). Is comorbidity with ADHD a marker for juvenile-onset mania? *Journal of the American Academy of Child and Adolescent Psychiatry, 36,* 1046–1055.

Findling, R. L., Gracious, B. L., McNamara, N. K., et al. (2001). Rapid, continuous cycling and psychiatric comorbidity in pediatric bipolar I disorder. *Bipolar Disorders, 3,* 202–210.

Findling, R. L., McNamara, N. K., Gracious, B. L., et al. (2003). Combination lithium and divalproex sodium in pediatric bipolarity. *Journal of the American Academy of Child and Adolescent Psychiatry, 42,* 895–901.

Geller, B., Cooper, T. B., Sun, K., et al. (1998). Double-blind and placebo-controlled study of lithium for adolescent bipolar disorders with secondary substance dependency. *Journal of the American Academy of Child and Adolescent Psychiatry, 37,* 171–178.

Geller, B., Craney, J. L., Bolhofner, K., et al. (2001). One-year recovery and relapse rates of children with a prepubertal and early adolescent bipolar disorder phenotype. *American Journal of Psychiatry, 158,* 303–305.

Geller, B., Craney, J. L., Bolhofner, K., et al. (2002). Two-year prospective follow-up of children with a prepubertal and early adolescent bipolar disorder phenotype. *American Journal of Psychiatry, 159,* 927–933.

Geller, B., Fox, L. W., & Clark, K. A. (1994). Rate and predictors of prepubertal bipolarity during follow-up of 6- to 12-year-old depressed children. *Journal of the American Academy of Child and Adolescent Psychiatry, 33,* 461–468.

Geller, B., Warner, K., Williams, M., et al. (1998). Prepubertal and young adolescent bipolarity versus ADHD: Assessment and validity using the WASH-U-KSADS, CBCL and TRF. *Journal of Affective Disorders, 51,* 93–100.

Kafantaris, V., Coletti, D. J., Dicker, R., et al. (2001). Adjunctive antipsychotic treatment of adolescents with bipolar psychosis. *Journal of the American Academy of Child and Adolescent Psychiatry, 40,* 1448–1456.

Kafantaris, V., Dicker, R., Coletti, D. J., et al. (2001). Adjunctive antipsychotic treatment is necessary for adolescents with psychotic mania. *Journal of Child and Adolescent Psychopharmacology, 11,* 409–413.

Kowatch, R. A., Sethuraman, G., Hume, J. H., et al. (2003). Combination pharmacotherapy in children and adolescents with bipolar disorder. *Biological Psychiatry 53,* 978–984.

Kowatch, R. A., Suppes, T., Carmody, T. J., et al. (2000). Effect size of lithium, divalproex sodium, and carbamazepine in children and adolescents with bipolar disorder. *Journal of the American Academy of Child and Adolescent Psychiatry, 39,* 713–720.

Kutcher, S., & Marton, P. (1991). Affective disorders in first-degree relatives of adolescent-onset bipolars, unipolars, and normal controls. *Journal of the American Academy of Child and Adolescent Psychiatry, 30,* 75–78.

Lewinsohn, P. M., Klein, D. N., & Seeley, J. R. (1995). Bipolar disorders in a community sample of older adolescents: Prevalence phenomenology, comorbidity, and course. *Journal of the American Academy of Child and Adolescent Psychiatry, 34,* 454–463.

Lewinsohn, P. M., Klein, D. N., & Seeley, J. R. (2000). Bipolar disorder during adolescence and young adulthood in a community sample. *Bipolar Disorders, 2,* 281–293.

McClellan, J., McCurry, C., Snell, J., et al. (1999). Early-onset psychotic disorders: Course and outcome over a 2-year period. *Journal of the American Academy of Child and Adolescent Psychiatry, 38,* 1380–1388.

Neuman, R. J., Geller, B., Rice, J. P., et al. (1997). Increased prevalence and earlier onset of mood disorders among relatives of prepubertal versus adult probands. *Journal of the American Academy of Child and Adolescent Psychiatry*, 36, 466–473.

Orvaschel, H., & Puig-Antich, J. (1987). *Schedule for affective disorder and schizophrenia for school-age children: Epidemiologic* (4th version). Ft. Lauderdale, FL: Nova University.

Pauls, D. L., Morton, L. A., & Egeland, J. A. (1992). Risks of affective illness among first-degree relatives of bipolar I old-order Amish probands. *Archives of General Psychiatry*, 49, 703–708.

Pavuluri, M. N., Graczyk, P. A., Henry, D. B., et al. (2004). Child- and family-focused cognitive-behavioral therapy for pediatric bipolar disorder: Development and preliminary results. *Journal of the American Academy of Child and Adolescent Psychiatry*, 43, 528–537.

Pavuluri, M. N., Henry, D. B., Devineni, B., et al. (2004a). Child Mania Rating Scale (CMRS): Development, reliability and validity. *Biological Psychiatry*, 55, S84.

Pavuluri, M. N., Henry, D. B., Devineni, B., et al. (2004b). A pharmacotherapy algorithm for stabilization and maintenance of pediatric bipolar disorder. *Journal of the American Academy of Child and Adolescent Psychiatry*, 43, 859–867.

Pavuluri, M. N., Henry, D. B., Naylor, M., et al. (2004). A prospective trial of combination therapy of risperidone with lithiumor divalproex sodiumin for pediatric mania. *Journal of Affective Disorders*, 82 (suppl. 1), 103–111.

Pavuluri, M. N., Henry, D. B., Naylor, M., et al. (2005). Divalproex sodium in pediatric mixed mania: A six-month open-label trial. *Bipolar Disorder*, 7, 266–273.

Pavuluri, M. N., Herbener, E. S., & Sweeney, A. J. (2004). Psychotic features in pediatric bipolar disorder. *Journal of Affective Disorders*, 80, 19–28.

Pavuluri, M. N., O'Connor, M. M., Harral, E. M., & Sweeney, J. A. (in press). An fMRI study of the interface between affective and cognitive neural circuitry in pediatric bipolar disorder. *Psychiatry Research: Neuroimaging*.

Pavuluri, M. N., O'Connor-Marlow, M., Harral, E., & Sweeney, J. A. (2007). Role of the affective circuitry during facial emotion processing in pediatric bipolar disorder. *Biological Psychiatry*, 62, 158–167.

Pavuluri, M. N., Schenkel, L. S., Aryal, S., et al. (2006). Neurocognitive function in unmedicated manic and medicated euthymic pediatric bipolar patients. *American Journal of Psychiatry*, 163, 286–293.

Rice, J. P., Reich, T., Andreasen, N. C., et al. (1987). The familial transmission of bipolar illness. *Archives of General Psychiatry*, 44, 441–447.

Schenkel, L. S., West, A. E., Harral, E. M., et al. (in press). Parent–child interactions in pediatric bipolar disorder. *Journal of Clinical Psychology*.

Spitzer, M. (1987). Clinical aspects and practical applications of DSM-III. *Psychiatrische Praxis*, 14, 212–217.

Strober, M., Morrell, W., Burroughs, J., et al. (1988). A family study of bipolar I disorder in adolescence: Early onset of symptoms linked to increased familial loading and lithium resistance. *Journal of Affective Disorders, 15*, 255–268.

Wagner, K. D., Weller, E. B., Carlson, G. A., et al. (2002). An open-label trial of divalproex in children and adolescents with bipolar disorder. *Journal of the American Academy of Child and Adolescent Psychiatry, 41*, 1224–1230.

Werry, J. S., McClellan, J. M., & Chard, L. (1991). Childhood and adolescent schizophrenic, bipolar, and schizoaffective disorders: A clinical and outcome study. *Journal of the American Academy of Child and Adolescent Psychiatry, 30*, 457–465.

West, A. E., Schenkel, L. S., & Pavuluri, M. (in press). Early childhood temperament in pediatric bipolar disorder and attention deficit hyperactivity disorder. *Journal of Clinical Psychology.*

Wilens, T. E., Biederman, J., Kwon, A., et al. (2004). Risk of substance use disorders in adolescents with bipolar disorder. *Journal of the American Academy of Child and Adolescent Psychiatry, 43*, 1380–1386.

Wilens, T. E., Biederman, J., Millstein, R. B., et al. (1999). Risk for substance use disorders in youths with child- and adolescent-onset bipolar disorder. *Journal of the American Academy of Child and Adolescent Psychiatry, 38*, 680–685.

Wozniak, J., Biederman, J., Faraone, S. V., et al. (1997). Mania in children with pervasive developmental disorder revisited. *Journal of the American Academy of Child and Adolescent Psychiatry, 36*, 1646–1647.

Wozniak, J., Biederman, J., Kiely, K., et al. (1995). Mania-like symptoms suggestive of childhood-onset bipolar disorder in clinically referred children. *Journal of the American Academy of Child and Adolescent Psychiatry, 34*, 867–876.

Youngstrom, E., Findling, R., Calabrese, J., et al. (2004). Comparing the diagnostic accuracy of six potential screening instruments for bipolar disorder in youth aged 5 to 17 years. *Journal of the American Academy of Child and Adolescent Psychiatry, 43*, 847–858.

Index

Labeling, 194
Lability, 19
Lamictal, 89, 92–93, 96, 97, 99
Laughing fits, 30
Learning ability, 26–27
Learning about bipolar disorder. See
    Information regarding bipolar disorder
Lecithin, 103
Legal issues, 153–154, 210
Lexapro, 88, 96, 99, 106–107
Light therapy, 105
Limit setting with your child, 78–79. See also
    Parenting
Lithium, 83, 89, 90–91, 96, 97, 98, 99
Living in the now, 126–127
Logical thinking, 17
Loving your child, 7, 144–146
L-tryptophan, 104

Maintenance treatment, 135–136. See also
    Treatment
Mania
    child- and family-focused cognitive-
        behavioral therapy and, 2–3
    decreased need for sleep, 31
    elated mood and, 18
    first medicine choices and, 88–102
    grandiosity and, 30
    medication options and, 97–98
    mixed with depression, 19
    mood regulation and, 119–123
    overview of, 15–16, 33
    subtypes of bipolar disorder and, 35
Manners, 78
Marijuana use. See Substance abuse
Marriage, 24–25, 172–177. See also Family
    conflict
Masturbation, 31–32. See also
    Hypersexuality
Meals, 18, 119, 164
Medical conditions, 40
Medication. See also individual names of
        medications
    brain functioning and, 74–75
    changing, 86
    common dilemmas regarding, 82–86
    complementary treatments to, 102–104
    developing a relationship with your doctor
        and, 58, 59
    FDA approval for children and, 85
    first treatment choices, 88–102
    forgetting to take, 109
    friends and, 231
    list of, 249–251
    management of, 109–110
    mood regulation and, 120–121
    multiple conditions and, 105–107
    overview of, 81–82
    paying for, 110–113
    Pediatric Side Effects Checklist (P-SEC),
        246–248
    privacy regarding, 110
    problems in, 107–109

reactions to that resemble bipolar disorder,
    40
recording information about your child
    and, 58, 59, 244–245, 246–248
routine and, 186
sleep patterns and, 118–119
stimulant medication, 38
stopping, 88
swallowing pills, 109
teleconferences between doctors and
    school personnel and, 255
types of, 87–88
when to consider a change in doctors and,
    70
while on vacation, 186–187
working with specialists and professionals
    and, 65
working with your doctor and, 61, 62
Megavitamin therapy, 104–105
Memory, 17, 26–27
Mental health parity, 111
Messiness, 31
Mighty-BD, 2, 5–7, 71–72, 239
Misbehaving, 19, 39
MITY-BD, 2, 5–7, 71–72, 239
Money issues
    babysitters or respite care providers and,
        177
    finding a doctor and, 51–52
    obtaining therapy and, 136–137
    paying for a therapist, 67–68
    paying for medication, 110–113
    paying for the evaluation, 45–46
    taking care of yourself and, 159–160
Mood. See also Anxiety; Depression;
        Irritability; Mania
    mixed, 19, 20, 35, 182
    mood charts and, 58, 121–123, 252. See
        also Charting information about your
        child
    overview of, 19, 30, 33–34
    regulation of, 4, 116, 119–123
Mood stabilizers, 88–102, 250–251
Mothers, 22–23, 24–25, 27–28, 154–160. See
        also Parenting; Parents
Motor skills, 17
Movements, involuntary, 107–108
Multi-Modal Integrated Therapy for Youth
        with Bipolar Disorder (MITY-BD), 2,
        5–7, 71–72, 239
Multiple disorders, 18, 105–107
Munchausen syndrome, being accused of, 23

Name calling, 79, 121
Narcissism, grandiosity and, 30
National Alliance on Mental Illness
    (NAMI), 50
Natural treatments, 102–104
Negative thoughts, 4, 116, 125–127, 149–
    150
Neuroleptic medications, 89, 93–94
Neurological evaluation, 44. See also
    Evaluation for bipolar disorder

About the Author

Mani Pavuluri, MD, PhD, is Associate Professor of Child Psychiatry and Founding Director of the Pediatric Mood Disorders Clinic and Pediatric Bipolar Research Program at the Institute for Juvenile Research, University of Illinois at Chicago. She is a widely cited expert on psychiatric disorders in young children and has been listed as one of "America's Top Psychiatrists" by the Consumers' Research Council of America and as one of the "Best Doctors in America" in Best Doctors, Inc.'s survey of physicians.